Managing Herpes

Managing Herpes

HOW TO LIVE AND LOVE
WITH A CHRONIC STD

by Charles Ebel

AMERICAN SOCIAL HEALTH ASSOCIATION
RESEARCH TRIANGLE PARK, NORTH CAROLINA

American Social Health Association, Research Triangle Park, NC 27709-3827

Design: Colleen Carrigan, Mills/Carrigan Design
Cover art: "To Choose the Uplifting" (oil on canvas)—Sue Sneddon
Illustrations: pp. 11, 27, 32-35—Mike Dulude
Photo credits: cover—Clear Light Studio; back cover—Les Todd

Library of Congress Catalog Card Number: 94-77927
ISBN 1-885833-03-2

CONTENTS

CONTENTS

CONTENTS

ILLUSTRATIONS

FOREWORD

There is a rich history behind these pages, a history that makes this work perhaps unique in the field of health education.

The genesis of the project goes back to the late 1970s. At that time, the medical and public health communities in this country were at last beginning to recognize the scope of the genital herpes epidemic that had been ongoing for some time. Genital herpes and its major complication, neonatal herpes, were being recognized more commonly by clinicians, yet laboratory assays to accurately diagnose the infection were not widely available and misinformation was widespread. Patients, meanwhile, urgently pressed for knowledge about a complicated viral infection for which there was no therapy.

At this time, Dr. King Holmes and I initiated a clinic at the University of Washington devoted to the study of genital herpes. As part of this program, we held an evening tutorial session one to two times monthly for patients and their partners. In addition, we started a telephone counseling service. Our own purposes at first were to screen and enroll individuals with herpes in our research studies. The service grew, however, and its staff soon found themselves faced with a great many questions that went beyond the limits of scientific knowledge.

The staff of the American Social Health Association, meanwhile, was wrestling with similar issues. ASHA had a 65-year tradition in public education on sexually transmitted diseases, and as the major national nonprofit organization in the field was increasingly overwhelmed with requests for herpes information. ASHA staff members Sam Knox and Carla Hines approached me with the idea of starting a nationwide consumer education group specifically directed at people affected by the epidemic. The program would be distinct in two ways: it would publish a newsletter devoted to the subject of genital herpes, directed primarily at those infected; and it would foster local discussion groups to assist people through face-to-face counseling. Each local chapter would be staffed by volunteers and affiliated with a volunteer health-care provider who would bring medical expertise to the chapter. Beginning in 1979, a scientific advisory committee of academic, industry, and government health-care professionals involved in the area of genital herpes was initiated to provide medical oversight to this national program, which became known as the Herpes Resource Center.

Over the past 19 years, the accomplishments of the program have been numerous. *The helper*, the newsletter that started the program, has become recognized as an authoritative, independent publication on medical, social, and psychological aspects of herpes simplex infections, and its success has been a model for other publications. The Herpes Resource Center also has hosted national conferences for medical practitioners, has worked with the news media, and has built a network of more than 100 local support groups. The chapters serve as local resource centers for patient information about HSV and other STDs. They operate local hotlines, help on referrals for specialized diagnostic services, and provide educational and psychological support for individuals needing to understand the complex biology of this infection. In addition, largely through individual donations, the program has sponsored postdoctoral fellowships for physician scientists to work in the area of genital herpes. In 1980, ASHA also initiated the National Herpes Hotline, which takes some 25,000 calls per year.

This book provides a further extension of the Herpes Resource Center's work and an outgrowth of the expertise it has established in this field. Charlie Ebel, who was the managing editor of *the helper* for over seven years, has become one of the most knowledgeable persons in the country on the issues of genital herpes. Over this period, I had the pleasure of watching his remarkable ability to synthesize complex scientific data into a readable style. What's more, his writing merges an understanding of the technical issues with an appreciation of the emotional aspects of genital herpes.

This book reviews an array of controversial medical issues, including diagnosis, transmission to partners, subclinical shedding, and alternative and traditional medical therapies. It is a unique contribution, and I am sure both the public and medical practitioner will find it invaluable.

LAWRENCE COREY, M.D.
SEATTLE, WASHINGTON

PREFACE

    At the National Herpes Hotline, the phone rings all day, every day. "Can you tell me if this is really herpes?" the callers want to know. "Do you think I got this from my lover?" "Is my doctor right when he says I'll have it for the rest of my life?" "Will I ever be able to date again?" "Can I have healthy children?"

    Since 1979, the American Social Health Association (ASHA) has been helping tens of thousands of people each year find answers to questions like these. Genital herpes, it seems, is not an illness that can always be resolved through a visit to the doctor or a course of treatment. It often looms much larger in the lives of those infected, complicating their most intimate relationships.

    ASHA, which has the goal of eliminating all sexually transmitted diseases, is the lone national organization that offers an outreach program specifically for people with herpes. Some 50,000 people yearly turn to ASHA for help, but with the number of new genital herpes infections estimated at half a million each year, these people represent only the tip of the iceberg. Many others don't know where to turn. So they carry the burden of nagging doubts and unanswered questions for months or years.

    This book draws on the experiences of those who have contacted ASHA for information or who have participated in surveys, support groups, and focus groups. To protect confidentiality, we have used fictional names. But the anecdotes you will find here are the stories of real people who have chosen to share them with us.

Likewise, the medical information and tips reflect the expertise of many fine scientists and health educators who have collaborated in guiding ASHA's herpes work over the past 15 years. This work includes local support groups and a quarterly journal, in addition to the National Herpes Hotline and educational material such as this book.

Two points of information about the format of the book are in order here. First, we're aware that choice of language can be a difficult issue. In writing about herpes, ASHA long ago abandoned terms such as "herpes victim," "sufferer" and "herpetic." Accordingly, we have chosen to use the term "people with herpes" through most of the text. There are, however, times when this label isn't quite as accurate or succinct as it should be. So you will also see the term "herpes patient" when we're discussing treatment options, for example, or communication with health-care providers.

Second, you will find a number of references in the text to a survey of people with herpes conducted by ASHA. In 1981 and again in 1991, ASHA surveyed a sample of several thousand readers of our quarterly journal, *the helper*. The results of the most recent survey were published in professional journals, and we have used them here to reflect a cross-section of opinion on several issues.

We hope this book offers some immediately useful guidance in managing genital herpes, and we hope also that it will prove a valuable source for future reference on herpes and other sexual health issues. But the best part is this: If you have further questions, we'll be here to help.

ACKNOWLEDGMENTS

In writing this book, I have drawn heavily on several articles published in the quarterly herpes journal published by the American Social Health Association (ASHA) and paraphrased the words of a long list of experts. I am particularly indebted to past and present members of ASHA's Scientific Advisory Committee on herpes, principally Lawrence Corey, M.D., Stephen Straus, M.D., Gray Davis, Ph.D., Zane Brown, M.D., Sevgi Aral, Ph.D., and Joan Wiebel, R.N.C. Other important influences were the writings of Gregory Mertz, M.D., Cal VanderPlate, Ph.D., Richard Keeling, M.D., Katherine Stone, M.D., Vincent Greenwood, Ph.D., Robert Bernstein, Ph.D., Rhoda Ashley, Ph.D., and Stephen Sacks, M.D. Special thanks to Anna Wald, M.D., of the University of Washington for her thorough review of the manuscript.

It's fitting also to acknowledge ASHA colleagues who helped to create our educational materials on herpes and researched or crafted some of the ideas presented here, among them Peggy Clarke, Diane Catotti, Burwell Ware, Melissa Peacock, Sara Townsend, Carolyn Mabry, and Nancy Herndon.

Last but not least, thanks to the stellar editorial and production crew who meticulously edited, typeset, indexed, and proofread two editions of this book: Sheryl Crabtree, Hilda Dawson, Kelli Edwards, Lisa Hyatt, Sandra Ackerman, Elinor Coates, and Charlotte Mizelle.

sexually transmitted infection. Growing up in American society, most of us come to view a sexually transmitted disease (STD) like gonorrhea or syphilis—or, more recently, herpes or human immunodeficiency virus (HIV)—as a strange and horrible event that happens only to those who have done something wrong. People who deserve trouble in their lives. People of bad morals. Attitudes about STDs vary depending on gender, race, religion, and other cultural factors, but very few of us can easily accept the fact that we have an infection spread through having sex. It's generally something about which we're taught to feel ashamed—or at least embarrassed.

Is this a reasonable attitude? Certainly few people would go out of their way to acquire an STD. Most of us would prefer to remain free of illnesses, whatever they might be. But the fact remains that all of us get sick during our lives. All of us are exposed to, and ultimately infected with, a host of bacteria and viruses that pose challenges to our health. Some of these germs are spread through the air or food or through contact with household objects that have been in some way contaminated. Some are spread through close physical contact with another person, including sexual contact.

Most of us are astonished to learn that infections spread through *sexual contact* are among the most widespread illnesses in our society. In fact, researchers believe that only the common cold surpasses STDs in the number of people affected. Each year, according to the U.S. Centers for Disease Control and Prevention (CDC), there are more than 12 million new cases of sexually transmitted disease. To breathe some life into that statistic, consider this: Every day you could fill Boston's Fenway Park to capacity with the number of Americans who picked up an STD in the previous 24 hours. You could fill every seat in this way, week in and week out, for years on end, because the STD epidemic shows no sign of slowing down.

When you think about it, the fact that STDs are so rampant shouldn't come as such a huge surprise. After all, people in all walks of life do have sex. It's as much a part of our biological make-up as eating and sleeping. And when we have sex, we sometimes pass a variety of common germs back and forth.

One of the most common, it turns out, is herpes simplex virus, the cause of genital herpes. This particular virus is a fact of life for at least 40 million Americans—about one in four adults.

It's normal to feel some embarrassment about getting any sexually transmitted infection, even to feel that this condition somehow separates you from your friends, or changes the way you will interact with them. But getting an STD is hardly a rare event. And as you can see, getting herpes puts you in rather large company.

All this is not to say that you don't have a right to your feelings. Herpes is for all of us an unwelcome guest, and one of the things about it that is so distressing is that it's probably a lifelong guest. Often the first questions we ask the doctor in that fateful office visit focus on getting rid of it. "What do we do about it? What drug can I take? What's the cure?"

The answer, as you probably know by now, is that medical science has no cure for genital herpes. There are a number of medications that can help to control herpes, although they cannot wipe it out entirely. Some people choose to rely on these to keep herpes under control, while others come to feel that they don't need any medicines. Researchers, of course, are still hard at their work. The next few years may see the release of new drugs and even vaccines for greater control of this infection.

In the meantime, it's important to remember that, with time, most people find herpes is not the catastrophe it seems to be at the start. The physical and emotional distress of herpes usually peaks early on, often in the first few months.

The experience of millions of people shows that herpes doesn't have to be—and usually isn't—a major, life-changing event. For many, it does require a process of adjustment—in our view of ourselves, in our relationships, and sometimes in the way we approach our physical health and well-being. The first step is to gain a better understanding about herpes and the issues it raises in our lives.

You've already taken it.

2

A VIRUS
IS A VIRUS
IS A VIRUS?

Genital herpes is caused by a virus—herpes simplex virus, or HSV for short. In order to understand herpes more fully, it's important to start with the big picture and go over some key facts about viral infections. This chapter doesn't deal directly with many of the practical issues you may be facing if you're just recently diagnosed with herpes. But stay with it: A grounding in some of the basics here may help you later as you try to answer some of your own specific questions about genital herpes.

You may or may not remember much about viruses from high school biology, but you've been coping with them for most of your life. There are literally hundreds of families of viruses and thousands of individual types. The "rhinoviruses," for example, are the frequent culprit in the common cold. Influenza viruses cause the respiratory ailments known as "the flu." And a host of "enteroviruses" cause the intestinal disorders that almost everyone copes with from time to time. Other infectious diseases caused by viruses run the gamut from measles to hepatitis to skin warts.

HERPESVIRUSES: THE FAMILY TREE

Some people find the term "herpesvirus" confusing. Spelled out as one word, "herpesvirus" actually refers to a *family* of viruses with certain traits in common. This family includes Epstein-Barr virus, the cause of infectious mononucleosis ("mono"); varicella zoster, the cause of chicken pox in children and "shingles" in adults; and herpes simplex, the cause of "cold sores" on the face as well as genital herpes. (See table below.) The recently discovered herpesviruses—HHV-6, HHV-7, and HHV-8—may cause illness in some people, but research on these is in its infancy.

HERPESVIRUSES

HERPES SIMPLEX VIRUS, TYPE 1	HSV-1
HERPES SIMPLEX VIRUS, TYPE 2	HSV-2
EPSTEIN-BARR VIRUS	EBV
VARICELLA ZOSTER VIRUS	VZV
CYTOMEGALOVIRUS	CMV
HUMAN HERPES VIRUS, TYPE 6	HHV-6
HUMAN HERPES VIRUS, TYPE 7	HHV-7
HUMAN HERPES VIRUS, TYPE 8	HHV-8

As you can see from this family tree, most of us have had dealings with at least a couple of herpesviruses by the time we reach adulthood. Almost all of us, for example, are infected with varicella zoster as children. We suffer through the usual drudgery of chicken pox—the fever, the sores—until we pull through and shake the infection. Similarly, many of us have experienced a bout with "mono" sometime in our teens or early twenties.

Like all other viruses, a herpesvirus makes its way in the world by living in healthy cells. Once it gets a hold in the body, it finds a way to invade normal cells and disrupt their usual functions. The virus uses the machinery of the normal cell to produce more copies of itself, a process called "viral replication."

Medical science has found ways to kill many types of bacteria and other disease-causing microbes. The drugs called antibiotics, for example, prevent bacteria from dividing and multiplying. Perhaps because many antibiotics are so effective, we have come to expect a pill that will rid the body of whatever troublesome infection we face.

But most viruses, unlike bacteria, defy treatment—they can't be "cured" in the way we think of using antibiotics to cure strep throat. Because viruses are able to find refuge inside normal cells, scientists have found it more difficult to stop viral infections. The classic example is the common cold or the intestinal virus that takes us to the family doctor looking for relief. The usual response goes something like, "It's probably just a virus—there's not much we can do except to let it run its course."

In reality, a virus doesn't simply "run its course," tiring out and quitting by itself. Rather, it's our set of natural defenses—the immune system—that finally halts the illness brought on by viral invaders. The process may take days or weeks, but with the most common viruses the immune system eventually wins out, and the virus is eliminated. End of story.

Unfortunately, with herpesviruses the story has another chapter. The catch is that the herpesviruses find a way to retreat from

well.

• A person with genital herpes caused by HSV-2 has sexual intercourse with a partner and spreads the virus, causing the partner to develop genital herpes.

• A person with HSV-1 cold sores performs oral sex on a partner, causing the partner to develop genital herpes sores. In this scenario, we have genital herpes caused by HSV-1.

The spread of herpes is a complicated subject, and it's discussed in more detail later. For now, the important point to remember is that HSV spreads through skin-to-skin contact, from an area where virus is present to a skin site that is susceptible.

Active and Inactive Phases: A Thumbnail "History"

What happens when HSV gets in your body? Once infected, the pattern and timing of events differ somewhat from person to person, but the basics remain the same. Once HSV gains a foothold, the virus begins replicating, invading the local nerve cells, and spreading. The defining event of infection is called latency—the virus's successful effort to set up a permanent base of operations. Having traveled the nerve pathways, HSV finds safe sanctuary in a nerve root called a "ganglion" (see illustration). In cases of genital herpes, HSV retreats to the sacral ganglion, located near the base of the spine. In oral-facial herpes, HSV finds its way to the trigeminal ganglion, near the top of the spine. In these ganglia, the virus remains inactive, or latent, for an indefinite period of time.

The appearance of signs and symptoms during HSV's initial invasion is a tricky issue. The process of infection and latency

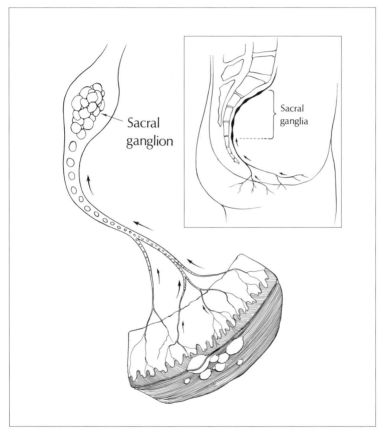

FIGURE 1. *HSV retreats along the nerves and finds sanctuary in the sacral ganglia, shown here.*

requires only a few days, and many people will experience obvious symptoms within the first 10 days. On the other hand, one's first encounter with HSV may cause changes so subtle that they aren't recognized. We'll discuss this in more detail in the next chapter.

Beyond the initial infection and establishment of latency, there is also the prospect of reactivation. When HSV is latent, various biological events can cause it to become active and begin traveling the nerve pathways back to the skin. There it can cause signs and symptoms once more (or perhaps for the first time).

How Common Is It?

Many people are shocked to learn how widespread herpes simplex is. Researchers estimate that between 50% and 80% of all American adults are infected with HSV-1. Many get an initial infection and have a bout with cold sores in childhood, and then have few or no recurrences of the infection in their adult lives.

Studies show that even if 80% of adults carry HSV-1, only a third of these individuals have ever had flare-ups with visible cold sores. HSV-1, then, is for the most part a commonplace and very benign infection. About 1 in 10 infected persons, or approximately 15 million, will experience recurrent oral-facial herpes several times per year.

HSV-2 is not quite so widespread, but it's hardly a rarity. Research data released in 1997 showed that 21.9% of Americans age 12 and older are infected with HSV-2, and the total number of people with genital herpes is estimated at more than 40 million.

If you're having trouble believing there are so many people with genital herpes, bear in mind that many of them don't know they have it. Researchers sometimes test blood samples in a population to find out what percentage have HSV-2. When they interview those who test positive, a surprising two-thirds or more say they have never had herpes. Then, when these apparently symptom-free individuals are questioned further, a majority will recall some minor symptoms that they had never thought of as genital herpes. The other group holds to its initial testimony: no history of genital sores or the like.

What makes one person react so differently from another when infected with the same virus? Some scientists guess that these result from individual immune responses, from the actual quantity of virus one is exposed to, or from the particular substrain of the virus involved. As yet, however, researchers can't fully explain the huge variability in herpes symptoms among equally healthy adults.

THE BOTTOM LINE

To cut through all the science, keep in mind a couple of very basic facts:

First, if you have herpes simplex, you have in your body a virus that operates in most ways just like dozens of other viruses you've carried around from time to time. The trouble with herpes simplex is that your immune system can't completely get rid of it. The virus can hide away and enjoy a lengthy stay through "latency."

Second, you're not alone. The majority of adults carry around herpes simplex, either type 1 or type 2—or both. They may not know it, because it may cause mild symptoms or no symptoms at all. But with latent infection, the potential for viral reactivation persists.

So, medically speaking, herpes is neither an exotic nor an especially dangerous infection in the vast majority of people. We're talking about a "garden variety" bug. No more, no less.

3

THE
FIRST EPISODE:
HSV'S INITIAL IMPACT

*"I was shell-shocked over having herpes anyway," says Erik. "But I
was also pretty sick. I had wet blisters on my genitals, I itched like I had
poison ivy, and I felt really run-down, too. It was almost like mono,
with a sore throat and swollen glands. I don't know whether I was
depressed or just sick, but I also felt listless—didn't want to do anything.
I just lay in bed most of the time, and missed a few days of work. Since
there wasn't any drug at the time, the only thing I could do for myself was
take warm baths a few times a day to relieve the itching."*

Many people infected with HSV either have very mild symptoms or no symptoms at all. But a significant number—perhaps
a third—will have noticeable symptoms of the infection. For
many, like Erik, the trouble begins with a very difficult period of
illness called the "first episode." This is likely to last longer and
to cause more discomfort and stress than any flare-ups that might
occur later.

THE IMMUNE RESPONSE

First episodes generally stir up considerable trouble because the invading virus has the element of surprise. Your body's defenses are down, and it takes a while before the immune system can identify the invader and refine its weapons to combat HSV. As it does, your immune response will succeed first in slowing the invasion and finally in forcing HSV to retreat from the field of battle.

Unfortunately, this doesn't happen overnight. The body's natural defense needs careful coordination among various parts of the immune system. These include the cellular immune response (the work of lymphocytes and macrophages) and the humoral immune response (antibodies). Using a combination of defenses, your body will try to kill virus as it moves from cell to cell, will get rid of cells already infected, and will try to protect cells that are still healthy.

As all this microscopic warfare is carried out, it may take several weeks before any progress can be made against the invading virus. But in the long run there is good news. After its initial struggle with HSV, your immune system will remain prepared for future encounters. For example, the body keeps on making the specific antibodies that cripple the virus, and they will work more quickly the next time HSV emerges from the nerve roots.

How long a first episode lasts will vary a great deal from person to person. Probably the important factor is your prior history with HSV.

Let's say that you've never had either HSV-1 or HSV-2 before. Through sexual contact you become infected with genital herpes caused by HSV-2. This is not only your first encounter with

HSV-2, it's your body's first glimpse of any sort of herpes simplex virus. So the virus is able to replicate and spread before the body can mount a fully effective counterattack. This is properly called a "primary first episode infection" or a "true primary." Because your immune system has no direct experience with HSV, the body is slow in marshaling its forces, and the signs and symptoms of infection are often troubling.

By contrast, let's say that you're one of the many people who was exposed to HSV-1 as a child and has been carrying the virus for years, whether you know it or not. At age 25, you become infected with HSV-2 through sexual contact and develop symptoms. Your immune system has seen HSV-1 before, but HSV-2 is a slightly different entity. Your natural defenses react promptly but aren't quite able to keep herpes in check. The result is a symptomatic "nonprimary first episode"—your first encounter with HSV-2. For simplicity's sake, we'll call these "first episodes." The symptoms, detailed below, can be severe, but not quite so severe as those of a "true primary."

As with many aspects of genital herpes, exceptions abound when it comes to describing symptoms, but the following descriptions sum up the experience of many genital herpes patients as they go through their initial outbreaks.

FIRST EPISODES (NONPRIMARY)

As we said earlier, the immune system that has already been exposed to HSV-1 may be able to keep the symptoms of HSV-2 to a minimum. If marked symptoms are going to emerge at all, they typically start within the first 10 days after exposure to HSV.

Often the first sign of trouble is a red spot or some other change in the skin on or near the genitals. Next comes the emergence of sores or "lesions." (The scientific literature on HSV uses the term "lesion" to describe any break or irregularity in the skin.) The classic lesions of herpes often resemble small pimples or blisters that eventually crust over and finally scab like a small cut. They also take the form of open sores ("ulcers" in the medical literature), particularly in women.

In first-episode genital herpes, lesions are likely to appear in men on the penis and urethra, the scrotum, the upper thigh, or around the anus. In women, they are commonly found on the vulva (lips of the vagina), urethra, cervix, and upper thigh, or around the anus.

Classic lesions that blister and crust over are often seen in first episodes, but signs of herpes come in a wide variety. They may be almost invisible to the naked eye or may look like a small pimple or insect bite, perhaps even going unnoticed. Then again, they may be large and obvious, superimposed on a patch of red skin. Sometimes sores will be extremely painful to the touch; sometimes they will not. Because of their varied appearance, herpes outbreaks sometimes are mistaken for heat rash, jock itch, or ingrown hairs.

When first seeing a doctor, people with first-episode genital herpes usually have several lesions in different places in the genital area. Almost half the time, these are followed by a new crop of lesions in the second week. All in all, first-episode lesions will cause pain or discomfort for an average of nine days and will take two to three weeks to heal fully. Lastly, as in the case of Erik, about one in six patients experiences more generalized symptoms, such as fever, malaise, headaches, and swollen glands, especially the lymph nodes near the groin. These generalized symptoms are more common in women than men.

"TRUE PRIMARY" FIRST EPISODES

Remember: A *true primary* first episode occurs when you've never had any type of herpes simplex before. With a "true primary," the pattern of events is similar to that of other first episodes, but the symptoms are generally a little worse. Herpes lesions will most likely appear in the same places, but there will be more of them and they will last longer. There is also a higher likelihood of a second wave of lesions starting in week two. Patients experience pain and discomfort for an average of 12 days, and herpes lesions usually require about three weeks to heal completely. A majority of people with primary genital herpes also will have the flu-like symptoms such as fever, swollen glands, and malaise. This, again, is especially true of women, and virus will be found on the cervix in most women.

Overall, in true primary cases there is more virus on the skin and it persists for longer periods of time, which raises the prospect of some other problems. One of these is the risk of getting herpes in other places—something known as "autoinoculation." The virus that's present on the surface of herpes lesions is contagious, not only to uninfected people but possibly to the patient as well.

Why? Primary and first-episode herpes cause such marked signs of illness because the immune system hasn't yet set up a solid defense for herpes simplex. And for the same reason, it's actually possible to spread HSV from one part of your body to

to get well and think things through before they're ready to resume sexual relationships.

WHAT YOU CAN DO

If you're experiencing your first bout with genital herpes, you're facing a host of issues and important personal decisions, such as whom to tell and how. Many of these questions are explored in detail in later chapters. The most immediate issues, meanwhile, are probably medical. Here is a brief list of steps that may help to keep the pain and anxiety of a first episode to a minimum:

- If you haven't already seen a doctor or other qualified health-care professional, do this right away. With symptoms such as fever, headache, and swollen glands, you have every reason to seek a professional consultation. In particular, find out for sure whether you do indeed have herpes. For this, you often need a laboratory test, since there are other infections that can cause symptoms similar to first-episode HSV. Some patients try to diagnose themselves and later regret it, always wondering if it's really herpes.

- A number of diagnostic tests are available (see Chapter Sixteen), but the most accurate remains the "cell culture." Find out which test your doctor has used, and, if possible, find out whether your symptoms are caused by HSV-1 or HSV-2.

• Discuss treatment options (which will be covered in Chapter Eight). Antiviral drugs such as acyclovir or related compounds, such as famciclovir or valacyclovir, can hasten the healing process in first episodes, sometimes by several days. Treatment also drastically reduces the duration of systemic complications, including meningitis.

• For help with the pain and discomfort of herpes lesions, consider taking a quick warm bath a couple of times a day. Some people say these provide excellent temporary relief. After the bath, be careful to dry the infected area gently with a soft towel, or use a hair dryer on the low setting. Keeping the area clean and dry not only relieves discomfort but can speed the healing process. The use of topical creams and ointments, on the other hand, can actually make matters worse. Avoid hydrocortisone creams and consult your doctor or pharmacist before using any over-the-counter products.

• Take good care of yourself. You need rest, good nutrition, and relaxation to get well fast. Having herpes may raise some emotional issues that cause additional stress; try to put these worries on hold. The bottom line is that you're sick and you will get better soon. It may be easier to tackle some of the emotional issues a little later.

Both medically and psychologically, the first episode is in many ways the toughest challenge that HSV poses. Getting through it in the most positive way requires a variety of resources. These include competent and sensitive medical care, solid factual information, and a sense of how herpes might affect important relationships. Beyond everything else, it's crucial to remember that the first episode is most likely the worst that HSV can throw your way.

4

RECURRENT GENITAL HERPES: THE LONG RUN

⟲

"It was about two months after my first outbreak," says Leslie. "Things were pretty much back to normal in my life, and I was hoping that I'd never have another flare-up. At the same time, I was really dreading the possibility that I might. Then one week I was working late a lot and having trouble sleeping. I ended up feeling kind of run-down, and a couple of days later, the herpes came back.

"I remember being really upset about that second outbreak, and obsessing about it, checking myself all the time. That probably made matters worse, but even so, the sores lasted less than a week. And other than some itchiness, I felt fine.

"It turned out that I had about four or five outbreaks that first year, all pretty much the same. I didn't do anything special about them, because they weren't that much of a bother. Later the outbreaks got milder, but I still had about the same number each year."

Like Leslie, if you're in the midst of a first episode, the very word "recurrent" may give you a feeling of dread. The prospect of "going through this again" is not a happy one. But don't think the worst: Recurrences of genital herpes are very different from first episodes and much less troublesome.

While Leslie's story is a familiar one, the specifics change for every individual. You may have only one or two herpes flare-ups in your whole life. You may have one or two each year. You may have a great many more. What happens in each case depends largely on a number of variables. Some, like the genetic make-up of your particular immune system, are completely beyond your control. But some you can influence by the way you manage your health.

LATENCY

To understand the mechanism of recurrent herpes, remember that HSV and other herpesviruses have the ability to hide away in the body. Immediately after you become infected, you may experience signs of illness (first episode) or may have no symptoms at all. Either way, your immune system will attack HSV and eventually force the virus to retreat.

Specifically, after the initial episode of genital herpes, HSV will move away from the skin surface and travel along the nerve pathways to the "sacral ganglia," the nerve roots at the base of the spine. There, it goes into an inactive phase in which it is protected from further attacks of the immune system. The virus's ability to hide in this way and establish a permanent presence is called "latency." During the latent phase, HSV does not replicate or move within the body. It's more or less in a state of suspended animation.

"REACTIVATION"

When latent HSV does become active, it begins to replicate. Traveling the pathways of the nervous system, the virus returns to the surface of the skin. There it can cause ulcers, sores, bumps, or other symptoms of genital herpes. This is often called "sympto-

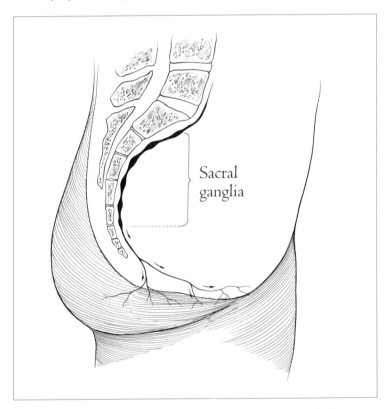

Sacral
ganglia

FIGURE 2. *When reactivated, HSV travels the nerve pathways back to the skin sur-face. Reactivation can cause virus to reach the skin at many different sites in the genital area.*

matic" or "recognized" reactivation, meaning that either the patient or the doctor has some physical evidence that HSV is again stirring up trouble.

Latent herpes simplex also can become active and travel the nerve pathways *without* causing signs and symptoms of illness. This phenomenon has been called a number of things, including "asymptomatic shedding," "asymptomatic reactivation," "subclinical reactivation," and "unrecognized" herpes. While there are

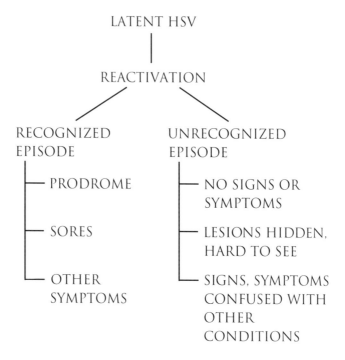

FIGURE 3. *Most people with genital herpes have both recognized and unrecognized reactivation.*

various terminologies describing reactivation without symptoms, the term "unrecognized herpes" is perhaps the most apt for three reasons: (1) Some lesions are overlooked because they occur in places we never look or can't see; (2) Some are mistaken for something else—an ingrown hair, for example; and (3) Some can't be seen at all with the naked eye.

WHEN YOU SEE IT, WHEN YOU DON'T

Scientists who study herpes simplex have used a variety of terms to describe its active phases, and many of these are confusing to those of us who don't have a technical background. Here's a brief primer on the most often-used terms:

Asymptomatic Reactivation, Asymptomatic Shedding:

These phrases denote the presence of virus on the skin or mucous membranes in the absence of symptoms. In strict usage, by the way, "symptoms" refer to any marker of disease—including subjective feelings such as burning or itching.

Subclinical Shedding:

The idea here is that herpes is likely to come to the attention of a health-care professional ("clinician") only if it causes a visible lesion ("clinical disease"). When it doesn't, it's called "subclinical." The most recent studies on viral shedding have tended to use this definition—the specific presence of a visible lesion—to distinguish between outbreak and non-outbreak.

Unrecognized Herpes:

The term used most often in this book takes a slightly different angle on the same phenomena, stressing the patient's ability or inability to perceive reactivation. By now, it's well documented that most people sometimes have viral shedding of which they're not aware. And sometimes it's difficult to know whether this shedding is accompanied by a small unseen lesion (subclinical) or by some pain or itch (symptomatic). The point is that very few people will always be able to recognize their signs and symptoms.

RECURRENCES WITH SYMPTOMS

Cases in which reactivation causes recognized lesions are usually called "recurrences" or simply "outbreaks." With these, people experience a wide range of symptoms, some of them very subtle. As with first episodes, there are certain classic symptoms worth mentioning.

Prodrome

First, many people notice an itching, tingling, or burning sensation in the genital area before they see any visible signs of illness. These sensations are called the "prodrome," and they can serve as a kind of early alarm system, warning that an outbreak may be on the way. Prodrome involves irritation along the nerves affected by HSV. Because nerve pathways connect in complicated patterns, this kind of irritation may lead to pain in the buttocks or the legs. Prodrome can last for several days but usually lasts less than 24 hours.

Other Signs and Symptoms

The prodrome is often followed by soreness or tenderness in a specific place, which in turn gives way to redness or skin irritation. Next, in many cases, ulcers or lesions resembling tiny blisters form on the skin. These can follow the same stages of healing described in Chapter Three, but fortunately, the lesions seen in a recurrence are usually fewer in number and heal more quickly. On average, any pain or discomfort is over within a week. Women tend to have more painful symptoms than men in recurrent herpes, but people of either sex very seldom have generalized symptoms such as fever, malaise, or fatigue.

Recurrent herpes usually affects the external genitals, less commonly reaching internal surfaces such as the cervix or the urethra. For example, unlike first episodes, recurrences produce evidence of virus on the cervix in only 12% of women, not the rate of more than 80% found in primary genital herpes.

We've already stressed that symptoms can vary a great deal from person to person. They can also change within an individual from one outbreak to the next, and certainly can change over long periods of time.

Genital herpes can cause very minor signs and symptoms that are easy to overlook. One example would be lesions that might occur on an internal part of the body such as the cervix or urethra. Not only are these out of sight, but they frequently clear up quickly.

There also are many cases in which herpes lesions look nothing like the classic blisters. They can instead be as subtle as a pimple, a small break in the skin, or a tiny area of redness. Sometimes herpes sores look like small linear fissures and are mistaken for a yeast infection. Sometimes they may fall at the site of a hair follicle and be mistaken for an ingrown hair. Another example is minor lesions around the rectum, which are hard to see and are commonly mistaken for hemorrhoids. (The wide variety of symptoms is the major reason that a visual diagnosis isn't always reliable.) In some cases, people experience prodrome and then have no lesions at all.

The skin lesions of genital herpes vary in appearance as well as in location. The following illustrations offer just a few examples of common sites for herpes recurrences. Lesions often are more subtle than those shown here.

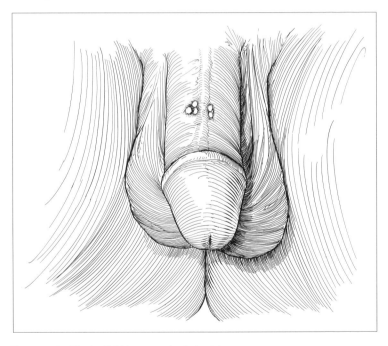

FIGURE 4. *Fluid-filled blisters on the shaft of the penis.*

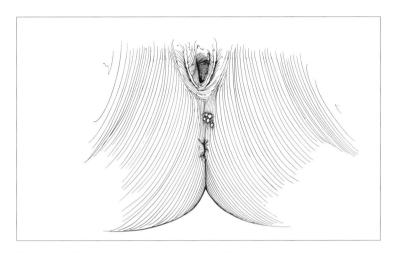

FIGURE 5. *Herpes lesions in the perineal area. (above)*
FIGURE 6. *Herpes lesions on the buttock near the anus. (below)*

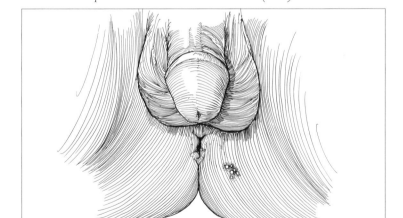

The pronounced lesions shown in Figures 4-6 can be found in both first-episode and recurrent genital herpes.

It's also worth noting that genital herpes symptoms don't always show up in the same place. A man might experience lesions on the scrotum the first several times he has an outbreak, for example, and then discover herpes lesions on the upper thigh the next time. The buttocks are another common nongenital site for herpes sores.

People sometimes find that the site of their outbreaks changes

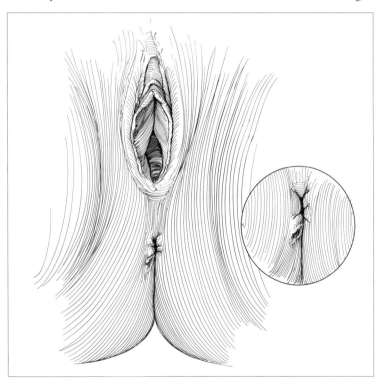

FIGURE 7. *A slight fissure (slit) near the anus, a common site for herpes lesions, which are sometimes mistaken for hemorrhoids.*

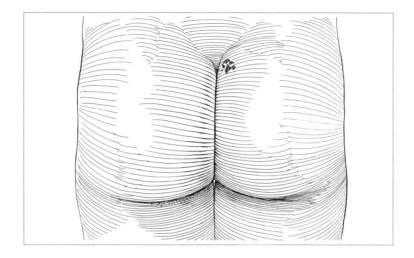

FIGURE 8. *Herpes lesions on the buttocks near the tailbone.*

over time, and they worry that the virus might show up anywhere. It won't. A genital herpes infection is limited by the nerve pathways connected to the sacral ganglion. With genital HSV, signs and symptoms may migrate a few inches here or there, but they will remain in the same general area below the waist. As noted earlier, there are instances in which herpes sores develop on the face, for example, during or after a troublesome first episode. These sores may result from "autoinoculation"; more commonly, though, they occur because a person has had a prior oral herpes infection. Don't jump to the conclusion that genital herpes has packed up and moved to the face on its own.

One further note on symptoms: A small number of people with genital herpes report pain or discomfort in the general area of the healed lesions *after* the normal symptoms of a recurrence have ended. The term sometimes applied to this condition is "post-herpetic neuralgia," meaning pain that extends along the course of one or more nerves. Post-herpetic neuralgia is frequently experienced by people with shingles, and has been studied best in that population. Unfortunately, however, there is very little research on HSV-related neuralgia: The frequency of this complication remains unknown, and there are no widely accepted guidelines on treatment. Experts in this area say that people experiencing pain or discomfort following an outbreak should regard HSV as being in its active phase during this time. They also suggest that analgesics such as aspirin or ibuprofen are probably the simplest remedies available for the pain; occasionally, more potent treatments are needed. For people in whom the pain is linked with frequent recurrences of genital herpes, there may be value in using a daily antiviral regimen (such as acyclovir) to suppress the outbreaks and thereby lessen the problem of repeated irritation to the nerves.

How Likely Are Recurrences?

It's difficult to predict the probability of recurrences in any individual case. There are, in fact, some people who never have anything resembling a herpes "outbreak," with blisters and the like. The latest research suggests that 10% to 30% of those with antibodies to HSV-2 recognize the infection: Equally important, among the more than two-thirds of seropositive individuals who are unaware of HSV infection, at least 60% can be taught to recognize recurrent symptoms. The bottom line: Most people with HSV-2 antibodies do have symptoms they can learn to recognize as herpes. In some cases, these might be marked outbreaks; in others, they might be minor irritations that could easily be overlooked.

These are large generalizations, taking into account all the millions of people for whom herpes symptoms will never be bothersome enough to spur a trip to the doctor. But the experts have more specific information when it comes to people whose first episode brought noticeable symptoms. Because these people often seek medical care, researchers have been able to run studies in which the patients are monitored for several years. These studies suggest that those with recognized herpes are almost certain to experience some type of recurrences, and those with longer lasting first episodes tend to have more frequent recurrences than those with milder first episodes.

Viral Type and "Sites of Preference"

Whether and how often you have recurrences depends to some extent on which type of HSV you have. If your primary episode is caused by HSV-1, for example, there is a 50% to 60% chance you will have a recurrence in the first year. By contrast, if the primary episode is caused by HSV-2, the chance of a symptomatic recurrence in the first year is 90%. And perhaps more importantly, people with genital HSV-2 are likely to have not just one but several recurrences in this and following years.

Why is this? Researchers don't fully understand it, but they know that type 1 and type 2 have definite "sites of preference." Scientists suppose that each viral type is triggered by certain events or chain reactions that may be specific to the body site where they're found.

In any case, HSV-1 causes the overwhelming majority of oral-facial herpes, and a person with HSV-1 latent in the facial area is much more likely to have recurrent outbreaks on the face than a person with HSV-2 in the same place. HSV-1 does account for about 30% of all genital herpes infections, and a first episode caused by HSV-1 is just as severe as that caused by HSV-2. But people with HSV-1 genital herpes are likely to have only a few outbreaks or none at all.

The site of preference for HSV-2 is the genital area. HSV-2 almost never recurs above the waist, but, as we've noted already, it's extremely likely to cause genital herpes outbreaks, not only in year one but in later years as well.

Long-Term Patterns

As with predicting the likelihood of recurrences, predicting their number and long-term pattern is very hard. One way that researchers have tried to get at this question is to interview people with genital herpes and ask them how many outbreaks they have over a 12-month period. For those with HSV-2, it seems that about a third has one to three outbreaks per year, another third reports four to seven, and the remainder has eight or more. The median rate is between four and five recurrences per year over the first two years after infection.

Over the same time period, people with symptomatic genital herpes caused by HSV-1 are less likely to have recurrences. Some experts, in fact, maintain that genital HSV-1 accounts for less than 5% of recognized herpes—the outbreaks that might prompt one to see a doctor or take medication.

Do outbreaks become less frequent after five years? Ten years? Do they become less severe? Medical science hasn't come up with conclusive answers to these questions. But recent studies on the long-term course of genital herpes suggest there is a slight decline in the number of recurrences for most people. However, herpes is highly variable from one person to the next, and some people continue to have frequent outbreaks for several years after acquiring genital herpes.

These observations are borne out by personal anecdotes. Unlike Leslie's experience at the start of this chapter, many people find that they have fewer outbreaks each year. Apart from their frequency, outbreaks also can become less severe. In the 1991 ASHA survey, 46% of the respondents said the frequency of their herpes outbreaks had decreased over time, while another 19% said the number of outbreaks per year stayed roughly the same. Only 12% cited an increase. The rest reported no predictable pattern.

Asked about the *length* of recurrences, 43% of respondents in the ASHA survey reported that outbreaks had become shorter over time, while 41% said they had remained the same. Only 3% said the length of recurrent flare-ups had increased. The remainder cited no predictable pattern.

REACTIVATION WITHOUT SYMPTOMS

For many years, scientists thought that HSV had basically two modes. One was the active phase, in which an infected person clearly had lesions or marked symptoms of some kind. The second was the inactive phase, in which HSV was out of the picture and of no consequence.

As they learned more about the virus, however, researchers

Scientists also have studied individuals who test positive for HSV-2 but have never recognized their signs and symptoms as herpes. These subjects were found to shed virus on roughly 3% of days, and while some become able to recognize herpes lesions, most episodes of viral shedding took place with neither signs nor symptoms present.

In summary, what's most remarkable about subclinical shedding is that it appears to follow the major patterns associated with recognized outbreaks: It often occurs immediately before or after symptoms appear; it's more likely with HSV-2 than HSV-1; and it produces quantities of virus sufficient to cause transmission. Moreover, subclinical shedding accounts for about one-third of all reactivation in those with recognized outbreaks and an even larger proportion of shedding in those with more subtle infections, so it's important to understand it. Researchers already have established that subclinical shedding, as well as shedding during recurrences, can be largely suppressed with medication. This is covered in Chaper Eight.

THE BOTTOM LINE

The next few chapters of this book offer many ideas on how to manage recurrent genital herpes. But there are a number of points we've already covered that are worth emphasizing:

> • If you have had a lengthy or troublesome first episode caused by HSV-2, you're probably going to have more flare-ups. These outbreaks will cause milder symptoms, and they'll usually last less than a week.

• Some people have only a few outbreaks each year, while others have many. The pattern is slightly different for everyone. If you have genital herpes caused by HSV-1, you most likely will be in the group that has fewer outbreaks—and less subclinical shedding, too.

• The symptoms caused by herpes outbreaks may also change over time. Sores might appear in one spot this month and several inches away three months from now. Some outbreaks may simply result in irritation or redness.

• You probably will have an early warning that an outbreak is on the way. It's that itchy or tingling sensation called the prodrome.

• The odds are that there will be several days out of the year when HSV reactivates but causes no symptoms.

• There is little hard evidence about what triggers outbreaks, but a great many people report that they associate certain stresses or behaviors with outbreaks. This will be discussed in Chapter Thirteen.

MANAGING HERPES

5

HOW DOES HERPES SPREAD?

"I was just diagnosed with herpes," says a caller to the National Herpes Hotline. "And I'm worried about giving this thing to someone else. I'm confused about how I got it, and I don't really know when I'm contagious."

Understanding how the herpes simplex virus operates and what you can expect it to do inside your body are crucial pieces of information. But equally pressing is the issue of *transmission*. People want to know how they got infected with herpes—when, and by whom, and in what precise way. And they also wonder when they're contagious now that they have it.

This is one of the most complex aspects of herpes and one that usually takes a bit of study to grasp fully. It may be necessary to read this chapter and the next a few times before the information makes complete sense, or before you can remember it all.

The first and most important rule to remember about herpes is that the virus can be spread from one person to another at any time when the virus is growing (replicating) on a skin surface or mucous membrane.

These active phases are often marked by signs or symptoms that herpes has flared up and reached the skin, such as the classic herpes lesions—obvious blisters that will take several days to go through a process of crusting, scabbing, and healing. Or they may be very mild symptoms that clear up in a couple of days. It's also possible that the changes caused by an active phase will be so subtle that you are totally unaware of them. This scenario will be explained more fully later in this chapter (see the section titled, "When No Symptoms Are Present").

The second rule to remember is that herpes is spread through *direct skin-to-skin contact* with an area where HSV is active. The most flagrant sign that herpes has become active is the presence of sores or some kind of lesion, however small, on the surface of the skin. We'll address this issue first.

WHEN SYMPTOMS ARE PRESENT

As an example, during your first recurrence, let's say you have two or three herpes sores on the genitals. The sores are, in effect, little colonies of virus, and as long as you can see them, you have significant amounts of HSV present on the surface of the skin. If you have sexual intercourse while the sores are present, it's likely that your partner's genitals would come into direct contact with these sores. That would give the virus a chance to spread to your partner's skin and take up residence there.

The risk of infecting another person begins with the itching or tingling feeling that you get right before an outbreak. If you notice any symptoms of recurrent genital herpes—even the prodrome—take it as a sign that the virus has found its way to the skin or to the mucous membranes usually affected. The risk continues as long as you notice *any* kind of symptom. If sores or other skin lesions are present, it's best to consider these contagious until they have completely healed. The tender new skin you see after a scab falls off might not be contagious, but caution is advisable: Subclinical shedding is more likely to occur within the first few days before and after an outbreak than at other times. And tender, newly healed skin also may be vulnerable to abrasion from vigorous sexual activity.

Herpes can be spread through other forms of direct skin-to-skin contact as well. Consider what can happen during oral sex. When a person with a cold sore on the lips has oral contact with a partner's genitals, the virus has an opportunity. Herpes can spread from the lips to the partner's genitals, causing genital herpes.

The direct contact that occurs during oral sex also can cause an infection in the facial area. Let's say a person engages in oral sex with a partner who has herpes sores on the genitals. Contact with those genital sores can give the virus a chance to spread to the lips, later resulting in a herpes outbreak in the facial area.

People can find all this a little confusing. They sometimes ask, for instance, "Now that I've got genital herpes, does it mean the virus is going to migrate all over my body and trigger cold sores on the lips?" Or they wonder if they're going to be spreading herpes when they touch someone or kiss someone. The fact is that herpes simplex will not relocate from your genital area to your facial area—at least, not without a lot of help. It can be spread from the genitals to a sexual partner's face in the way we just described, but it doesn't get up and move all by itself. Remember the rule of thumb: Herpes is spread through direct skin-to-skin contact with an area where virus is active on the skin.

You may be wondering why herpes seems to take hold only in

the genital region or around the mouth. Like many viruses and bacteria, HSV prefers warm and moist environments. And the tissue of genital skin like that of the vulva or penis offers the virus a suitable entryway. So do soft, moist surfaces such as the vagina, cervix, anus, and mouth. The thicker, tougher skin on the arms and legs, by contrast, is generally not hospitable to germs and viruses such as herpes simplex. If by chance herpes simplex virus is deposited on these parts of the body, it usually withers before it has a chance to find the nerve pathways and go about the complex business of making its permanent home.

Notice the word "usually" in the last sentence. There are some cases where herpes does penetrate the tough skin of the hands or the chest, for example. But in these instances the process of transmission is helped along by some damage to the skin in question.

A good illustration of this principle is a phenomenon called "herpes gladiatorum"—what some might call "wrestler's herpes." In a number of cases, high school or college wrestlers have developed herpes sores on the chest or arms in the aftermath of a wrestling tournament. Why? Wrestling involves rolling around on the mat and grabbing the arms and torso of the opponent, all of which can be abrasive to the skin—even thick skin. Add to this the fact that wrestlers spend a good deal of time in tight embraces, and you can see that direct contact with a cold sore might give HSV a chance to spread from one wrestler to another.

This happens only rarely, and the circumstances under which it has occurred sometimes involve a wrestler who is particularly contagious because he is having a first outbreak or a "true primary" episode of type 1 herpes on the face. During this kind of outbreak, unusually large amounts of virus might be present on the surface of the skin or in saliva.

Another scenario in which herpes can spread to thicker skin is "autoinoculation." As described in Chapter Three, this occurs when someone touches a herpes sore—on the genitals, let's say— and then ends up sometime later with a herpes outbreak on the tip of the finger. The route of transmission is clear. Active virus from a sore found its way to the finger when the person touched or scratched the sore. The virus then managed to find some portal of entry—a cut or scrape, for example—so that it could travel the nerve pathways and set up shop in a different location, most commonly moving from the genitals to a finger or onto the face. Autoinoculation seems to be most common when the site of new infection is another mucous membrane. (Sometimes people get herpes sores in the eyes, a subject discussed in Chapter Fifteen.)

To keep this in proper perspective, don't forget that autoinoculation is relatively infrequent, and some of it results from contact with herpes lesions on the face. Researchers say that it occurs almost exclusively during first episodes or true primary cases, when there are lots of sores and an unusually high dose of virus on the skin. It's estimated that autoinoculation occurs in about 10% of first episodes, but it's uncommon with recurrent genital herpes. The reason is that over time the body develops a strong immune response to the virus.

To sum up, the best advice is to regard the presence of prodrome, sores, or any potentially herpes-related lesion as a sign that the virus is active and could be spread. Any kind of direct skin-to-skin contact with the sores or lesions creates a risk for the spread of the virus, but it's usually *sexual* contact—genital-to-genital, oral-to-genital, or oral-to-oral contact—that causes new infections.

WHEN NO SYMPTOMS ARE PRESENT

Unfortunately, the virus's active phase is not always marked by the presence of signs and symptoms. Chapter Four describes the phenomenon of unrecognized herpes, in which herpes reactivates and travels to the skin without setting off the usual alarm system. It's now clear from a number of studies that herpes can be spread at these times, in a process called asymptomatic or subclinical transmission.

These are troublesome facts of life for people with herpes, because they complicate the issue of protecting a sexual partner from infection. Nevertheless, there are a number of ways to approach this problem of unrecognized herpes, and the best way to begin is by understanding more about how it works.

In a general sense, unrecognized or subclinical shedding is somewhat similar to regular outbreaks: While herpes is in its latent phase, some event triggers a flare-up. HSV travels through the nerve pathways to the area where it usually causes symptoms, and some virus finds its way to the surface of the skin. Meanwhile, the immune system comes into play and thwarts the virus, stopping the flare-up before any major lesions appear—but unfortunately *not* before there is risk of transmission.

Where is the subclinical shedding likely to occur? In most cases, HSV can be expected to travel the same routes it does during a regular flare-up, and virus might reach the skin anywhere in the genital area, including the sites where you normally have signs and symptoms during a noticeable outbreak. In particular, subclinical shedding is likely on the vulva, perianal area, and cervix in women, and the penis and perianal area in men.

Subclinical shedding is not constant but periodic. As was

explained in Chapter Four, rates for viral shedding often decline slightly over time, and subclinical shedding ultimately may occur on a handful of days per year. The hard part is that you won't know which days these will be. So when it comes to protecting a sexual partner, this is an issue that requires you to talk things through and make certain decisions as a couple.

In the category of good news to report, researchers have found antiviral therapy has the same effect on subclinical shedding that it does on outbreaks. In particular, a daily dose of antiviral medication brought about a 94% reduction in shedding in one study. Therefore, those at high risk of shedding may benefit from therapy.

OTHER ISSUES FOR TRANSMISSION OF HSV

An important concern for couples who would like to have a child is the issue of managing herpes during pregnancy and birth. In some cases, HSV is transmitted to a baby at the time of delivery if the mother has active herpes in the birth canal at delivery. This is a very rare event among the tens of millions of women who have genital herpes, and there are well-known precautions that can prevent it in most cases. All the same, herpes infections in a newborn can be life-threatening, and expectant parents often have very specific questions about what they need to do to ensure a healthy birth. They also wonder about the risk to an infant in the home if one or both parents have recurrent genital herpes. We've attempted to answer these questions in detail in Chapter Fourteen.

Another frequent question centers on the spread of herpes from *things* rather than from people. Can you get herpes from a toilet seat, for example, or a dirty towel? The basic answer on the risk of getting herpes from inanimate objects like these is something along the lines of "generally impossible." The main reason for this goes back to our earlier discussion about transmission, about skin-to-skin contact, and about the likely places where herpes can take hold. If you rubbed a herpes sore against a towel, for instance, some of the herpes simplex virus could be deposited onto the towel. The virus may persist outside the body for several hours, but almost immediately it begins to shrivel, losing its ability to invade and colonize new cells.

Now take the example of the toilet seat and follow the rules of transmission. In order to spread herpes, a person has to be infected, to have active herpes, and to have virus present on the skin. Furthermore, the skin in question would have to come into contact with the surface of the toilet seat. Since people generally do not rub their genitals against toilet seats, a person would have to have active herpes on the back of the thigh in order to place virus on the seat. This is an unlikely place to have an outbreak.

Next, within a short time, a second person would have to sit on the same seat, making contact with the seat in exactly the same spot, thereby coming into contact with the now-withering herpes virus. And would the virus find a hospitable environment there on the back of the thigh? Probably not. The skin there is thick, making it an unlikely target for HSV.

Researchers do acknowledge a theoretical risk of spreading herpes in other ways. A damp towel shared by two people showering together, for example, could hypothetically provide a means for the spread of herpes to the genitals if one person were having an outbreak and rubbed the towel on the site of infection before passing it to the partner. Experts disagree about whether herpes is ever *really* spread in this way, but because it's theoretically possible, researchers agree on common sense precautions. During active phases, they suggest, don't share towels, underwear, or other objects that come into contact with herpes sores. In cases of facial herpes, the items to avoid sharing during active phases would be cups, toothbrushes, and razors. And if you touch a herpes lesion with your finger, take the precaution of washing your hands right away. Soapy water kills the virus.

PEOPLE WITH HERPES are likely to have a number of worries about spreading the infection to other people. It's natural to have these concerns. But sometimes people will become obsessed with risks that are either very remote or completely nonexistent. So, to put things in perspective, here are some overall guidelines.

- The greatest risk for spreading herpes comes when you have a type of herpes symptom—no matter how slight— and your partner's skin comes into direct contact with that area during sex. Avoiding this kind of contact is the first concern.

- If you have recurrent genital herpes, you will want to talk with your lover about the risk of subclinical transmission when you have sex during the times between outbreaks. See Chapter Eleven for a full discussion of the different approaches that people take to prevent the spread of herpes in sexual relationships.

- If you're having your first-ever outbreak of genital

herpes (or facial herpes), it's wise to be extra-cautious about hygiene. Avoid touching herpes sores, and if you do touch them, wash your hands right away with soap and water. Soap will kill the virus.

• If you are pregnant and you or your partner has a history of genital herpes, it's very important to inform your physician or midwife about this part of your medical history. If genital herpes becomes active at the time of delivery, your provider may need to take special precautions to protect your baby.

• If you have a newborn in the household, take care to see that the child does not come in direct contact with herpes lesions. It wouldn't be wise, for example, to kiss anyone if you have a cold sore on the mouth. This is an especially important rule with infants.

The most critical issues for preventing transmission of HSV center on your sexual relationships. These will likely be among your biggest concerns as you adjust to life with the herpes simplex virus.

6

WHO'S TO BLAME?

"It was a mystery," says Julia. "I remember being diagnosed with
herpes and wondering where I got it. I didn't have a clue. I hadn't slept
with anyone in a couple of months. So I called the two people I'd been
with before that, and both said they'd never had herpes. They thanked me
for telling them about it. That was it. I never figured it out. And I
never knew if I gave herpes to anyone else. I still wonder."

If you've just experienced your first outbreak of genital herpes, you, too, may be asking the question: Where did I get this?

Given that genital herpes is a sexually transmitted disease, it's
natural for people to scrutinize their current sexual relationships
in the search for an answer. Often they seek to blame a current
partner for infecting them, especially if it's someone they've
known only briefly. If they have been intimate with one person
for a long time, they sometimes come to believe that this partner
has recently had an affair, developed herpes as a result, and kept it
a secret. Whatever the scenario, suspicion and anger are common
elements, and they're often directed at a person's current lover.

Are these suspicions likely to be well-founded? It is possible
to get a genital herpes infection from one's current sexual partner,
but this is not always the correct explanation. Julia's story doesn't

offer enough detail for even an educated guess, but with a little room for embellishment we can suggest at least three possible scenarios:

"It Had to Be You"

Julia is single and dating, having recently broken off a relationship of two years with Jim. She's currently seeing Mark off and on, and two months ago she slept with him a few times. Later she developed a rash of blisters and went to the doctor, who now has diagnosed her with genital herpes.

Can Julia legitimately blame Mark? The circumstantial evidence is fairly damning, but in this example Julia actually had acquired herpes from her earlier boyfriend, Jim. Neither of them knew he had it, because he was one of those many millions who carry HSV-2 and never realize it. She never knew she had gotten it, because she had no obvious symptoms when she was first infected.

Now, years later, something has triggered a reactivation of the latent HSV. Julia has symptoms, and she's blaming Mark.

"It Had to Be Infidelity"

Let's keep two of the players, but change the details of the story:

Julia has been living with Mark for almost a year. She gets genital herpes symptoms and is diagnosed with it. She wants to blame Mark and so confronts him.

Mark says he doesn't have herpes—never had any STD or anything vaguely resembling herpes. Just as Julia suspects him,

Mark now begins to suspect her. He knows that he hasn't been intimate with anyone else for more than a year. Now suddenly he is accused of having herpes. So he wonders if Julia has recently had an affair, has picked up this infection, and is simply afraid to admit it.

Well, Mark is wrong. It turns out that Mark does have herpes and did infect Julia. It's just that he didn't know he had it. He's one of those people who has very mild symptoms and isn't aware that anything is wrong. For all practical purposes, he's being completely honest and above-board. But he does have herpes. And now Julia does, too.

"A Long Story"

Let's try one more variation:

Having broken off a relationship with Jim a year ago, Julia moves in with Mark. Two months later Julia comes back from the doctor with a diagnosis of genital herpes. She blames Mark; Mark blames her. Accusations of infidelity fly. Mark denies any history of herpes.

Then suddenly Mark, too, gets herpes. Julia is now fully convinced that she was right to blame him all along. Mark is equally convinced that Julia is at fault.

As in the first scenario, Julia actually had picked up herpes from her earlier relationship with Jim. But things have gotten really complicated now. Julia never knew she was infected until she just recently had her first outbreak. Meanwhile, she had infected Mark.

Everybody has herpes, and it all started with Jim.

IS REAL LIFE like this? It isn't always, but it can be. Each of these scenarios is quite plausible.

If there is appeal in a guessing game, tracing genital herpes infection can be among the most challenging of mysteries. Countless people with herpes have puzzled over the spread of HSV and posed hard questions: How could this have happened to me? Are you sure it wasn't a toilet seat? Who was the culprit? Was my spouse unfaithful? Did my lover know he had herpes and deliberately keep this from me?

For the most part, the questions cannot be answered. HSV, it turns out, is a very crafty virus. Trying to figure out how it spreads raises a host of complicated issues: signs and symptoms, viral type, previous sexual history, prior infection with HSV, and so on.

The fictional scenarios presented here offer a glimpse at three critical reasons why it's hard to know who is to blame.

The first reason is that *you can have herpes and never know it.* Earlier chapters have gone into some detail about the evidence that more than two-thirds of all people with HSV-2 infection deny having genital herpes when asked. Some probably never have symptoms. Some have mild symptoms they never recognize as herpes. But either way, a large number of people get herpes and never know it, never think about it—never have any reason to talk about it or take precautions.

The second reason is that *you can get herpes and carry it around for months or years before you finally have a recognized outbreak.* Researchers believe that something like one in four people seeking care for their first outbreak have actually had herpes for some time. It's possible to have a very mild first episode and to assume that it's something else—a yeast infection or an allergic rash, for example. Then, seemingly out of nowhere, the person with a mild or unrecognized infection can one day face a troublesome outbreak and wrongly assume that genital herpes is a new problem.

The third reason, and major confounding factor, is that *you can spread herpes even when you don't have symptoms.* Furthermore, herpes can be spread by those who never have symptoms. In reality, whether they have symptoms they recognize or not, these individuals do have reactivations of genital HSV. So there are times when virus is present on the skin. And that raises the possibility of spreading it to someone else. People who know they have genital herpes usually take some precautions to protect sexual partners, at least during known outbreaks. People who are unaware they have it often don't take precautions.

Of course, subclinical transmission is a risk even for people with outbreaks that they do recognize as genital herpes. Sometimes a person might be careful to refrain from sex when symptoms are present but be unlucky enough to spread HSV to a partner during a period of viral shedding between outbreaks.

If all this seems a little overwhelming, be aware that it's overwhelming for almost everyone—including highly skilled medical professionals. If you're trying to pinpoint the source of your herpes infection, you may well run into some dead ends. And it's probable that your health-care provider won't be able to solve the mystery either.

Is there any way to know for sure? Can you get special tests that pinpoint the source? The path is laid with pitfalls, but there are some facts you can probably establish with the help of a medical professional. You may, for example, be able to make a pretty good guess as to whether you are having a true primary, a first episode, or a recurrent episode. The clues to be assessed include testing for antibodies in some cases as well as the symptoms you're experiencing: Do you have lots of herpes sores? Is it taking them more than two weeks to heal? Do you have fever, swollen glands, or other "systemic" symptoms of a first episode?

But all these clues won't necessarily tell you the source of your herpes infection. As the fictional scenarios at the beginning of this chapter suggest, a lot depends on your own sexual history and a host of factors too complicated to explain in a book of this size. The moral is this: Don't be too quick to judge the situation. Figuring out the source of a herpes infection can stump even the best medical detective.

What's more, even if you are fairly sure about how you got herpes, it can be very wrong to assume that the partner in question was acting irresponsibly. There are indeed some people who know that they have herpes and who withhold this information from sexual partners. But there are many more who have no idea they themselves are infected, much less that they might be putting you at risk. In the end, understanding and forgiveness are likely to give you more comfort than blame or vengefulness.

7

PATIENT AND PROVIDER

"My diagnosing doctor was rude and insensitive," says Trish. "He seemed unconcerned about my condition and said there was nothing I could do except go home and wait until the flare-up faded and went away. He said most people just see it as an annoyance. I was devastated."

Even if you normally get along well with your doctor, a diagnosis of genital herpes can complicate matters. People with herpes commonly report frustrations and complaints about their health-care experiences. It's important to be aware of some of the potentially tricky issues in order to continue a positive working relationship with your chosen medical professional.

If there are troubles, they often start with the visit in which herpes is diagnosed. The diagnosis itself is tough to hear and tough to deliver. And the discussion that follows often fails to meet expectations on both sides.

From the patient's point of view, it's often devastating to learn that the illness at hand is caused by a sexually transmitted infection. Worse still, it's a viral infection and will remain for life. This news raises a great many questions about herpes itself and about its potential impact on important relationships.

The medical information alone is complex. The first several chapters of this book, for example, cover most of the basics. But how many doctors have the time to cover those topics on a first visit, especially if they haven't had the chance to schedule an extended session? Beyond this, patients can bring up emotional issues for which the health-care professional may not have ready answers. "What will this mean for my sex life?" "How can I tell my lover?" Some of the questions cannot be answered in simple black and white.

From the provider's point of view, time and the patient's emotions are the constraints. Health-care professionals often say they do their best to counsel patients on the key points but that patients' feelings of anger or disbelief sometimes stand in the way. A patient might be too upset to take in a lot of medical information—or might not remember many details later even if they were covered in a counseling session. Plus, with a waiting room full of patients, there isn't time to say or do everything the health-care provider would like. Sometimes the best solution seems to be scheduling a follow-up visit. Even then, however, patients can leave unhappy.

There is also the problem of unrealistic expectations. We often seek health care assuming that all questions can be answered and all symptoms can be cured. But in reality medical professionals are not all-knowing or all-powerful, and herpes may force the issue. Faced with questions like "Where did I get this?" the health-care provider may well have to say, "I don't know." Rightly or wrongly, this can lead to feelings of frustration and helplessness in the patient. And when it comes to the emotional issues, providers may lack both the time and the specific training required.

We know from interviews and from surveys that large numbers of people with herpes voice complaints about their first visit and about the health-care provider who first diagnosed them. In ASHA's 1991 survey, more than half rate this provider as "poor" or "fair" when asked specifically about the provider's performance in answering questions, giving treatment information, offering emotional support, and discussing a patient's sex life.

Worse still, sometimes patients say that their providers make them feel ashamed about having herpes and make remarks that assess blame—for example, comments like "You now have to pay the consequences for what you've done." Another frequent complaint, voiced earlier from Trish, is that providers overlook the importance of leaving patients with a sense of hope or empowerment; instead they may seem to be saying, "There is nothing to be done." Either kind of experience can have the effect of closing the door on further discussion of herpes. It can keep patients from asking the questions they need answered, getting treatment for current or future outbreaks, and getting advice they may want on a fairly intimate matter. It sets a negative tone that is hard to change. As one support group leader comments, "People's attitudes during their initial bout with herpes are formed in the first few days and are shaped by how they're told."

If you have had a frustrating experience with your provider, you may be tempted to give up on medical professionals and turn inward. It's important to remind yourself, however, that you don't have to shoulder the burden of genital herpes alone. Strained relationships between the patient and the health-care provider often can be repaired. And if they can't, there is always the option of looking for a "second opinion." A great many patients

tions and concerns from time to time. You should feel entitled to raise them. People who take charge and get the answers they want seldom look back and regret it.

Even if you've had one bad experience regarding care for genital herpes, you may choose to keep the door open. Consider making one more appointment to discuss your concerns.

If you feel it's time to look elsewhere for medical care, physicians with specialty training in gynecology, urology, dermatology, and infectious diseases may have more experience or technical training on herpes. A family practitioner or other primary care physician, on the other hand, may offer better counseling or emotional support. Much depends on the individuals involved. You may be able to get a list of referrals from your local medical society or from a local herpes support group. If you have a university medical center or teaching hospital nearby, you can also reach the department dealing with "infectious diseases" and ask for a herpesvirus or STD specialist.

WHAT YOU CAN DO

- Inform yourself about herpes and make a list of the questions and concerns you need to raise with a healthcare professional. Many people find it's a good idea to bring the list (mentally or in written form) when you have the medical consultation.

- It may take persistence to get the answers you need, but don't be afraid to ask your provider for help. Knowledge and emotional support are tools that can help put you back in control. If you have trouble broaching the subject, you might take a few minutes to ponder and rehearse a script. You might say, for example, "I feel awkward bringing this up, but I've had a history of genital herpes and there are some things that I've been wanting to get professional advice on." If the questions include sexual matters, you might arrange to bring your partner along when you see the doctor.

• If you're interested in treatment, ask the provider to explain your options. This, too, can be a way to gain some control over herpes. Don't let yourself feel cut off from treatment just because your provider didn't bring it up the first time. "I realize that doctors don't always choose to treat genital herpes with medication," goes one typical script, "but I'm really having trouble with this and I want to know what the options are."

• Some herpes patients say they have established rapport with one provider but dread having to see other members of the practice for herpes flare-ups. For some it's a question of experiencing the awkwardness all over again. If you're served by a group practice of some kind, you may want to discuss the problem of continuity in your care for genital herpes, at least for the first year.

• If what you need is primarily emotional support, be realistic about what your medical professional can offer. Depending upon your personal situation, you may be best served by going to a support group, seeking out a friend or counselor, or looking to other resources. There is a list of ideas at the end of this book.

For some, these suggestions may beg the comment "easier said than done." Establishing good communication about herpes often takes a dose of hard work for both the patient and provider. Most experts stress three general points above all: Inform yourself; communicate your concerns and questions to your healthcare provider in an organized way; and don't be afraid to seek a second opinion if you're totally unsatisfied. The work might be hard, but it's a prescription you can write yourself.

8

TREATMENT
OPTIONS

"My outbreaks were frequent and troublesome," writes Teri. "It wasn't so much because of the sores, which cleared up quickly, but because of symptoms like headache, eye irritation, and muscle aches. It was like having the flu about once a month.

"I finally went to my gynecologist and went on a course of drug therapy that has changed my life. I take medication every day, and now I'm symptom-free, in spite of a very stressful, demanding job and an active sex life.

"So far, so good, I guess. But I don't like the idea of being so dependent on a drug and having to take it every day. Is this really safe over the long term? What are my choices?"

Like many other viral infections, genital herpes can be treated with various medications. There isn't yet a cure in the way that antibiotics can knock out a specific kind of bacteria, for instance. Once a person is infected, HSV will establish latency and remain in the nerve ganglion for life. But several medications can ease the symptoms of herpes, and may help to stop outbreaks altogether for as long as the medication is being taken.

Three prescription medicines are currently approved by the U.S. Food and Drug Administration for treatment of genital herpes. The best known and most widely prescribed is acyclovir. Sold under the brand name Zovirax® since 1982, acyclovir is now available as a generic. It's actually a rather remarkable drug—one of the first ever produced to be effective against a virus without being toxic to normal cells. The scientist who led its development, Gertrude Elion, received a Nobel prize for her research.

Acyclovir works by attacking the virus's ability to reproduce and spread. Like other viruses, HSV can move from cell to cell in its active phase, colonizing the cells as it goes and using them to create more virus. At the molecular level, the key to this process is the virus's genetic assembly instructions, or DNA (deoxyribonucleic acid). Acyclovir substitutes itself for one of the building blocks of the viral DNA, and in doing so fools the virus into accepting an impostor. Once acyclovir has slipped into the machinery of the virus, the DNA chain comes to a halt.

For the patient taking the medication, this translates into a win over HSV, as the virus eventually can be eliminated everywhere but the nerve ganglion, where it always finds safe haven between active phases. In practical terms, a patient with a nasty first episode might normally have to wait three weeks before the skin lesions are healed and things have returned to normal. With acyclovir treatment, the length of the outbreak might be cut significantly.

How significantly? This depends on the patient, the type of symptoms, the formulation of the drug, and how quickly the drug is administered. Just for the record, acyclovir has its strongest effect when taken intravenously. Generally, however, IV treatment is reserved for rare herpes complications or very severe cases. Oral acyclovir, in the form of capsules or tablets, is also very effective and is widely used for genital herpes. A weaker formulation of the drug is the topical ointment. This compares poorly with oral medication and is not recommended for genital herpes.

In addition to acyclovir, people with herpes have a choice between two newer antivirals. Both of these are "prodrugs," which means that they have a kind of two-staged delivery. Stage one is a compound that's taken into the body and easily absorbed. In stage two, the compound is converted by the body to an active medication.

One of the new prodrugs is marketed by acyclovir's maker, Glaxo Wellcome. Called valacyclovir (brand name Valtrex®), this drug converts to acyclovir on ingestion. This process has the advantage of being able to get higher levels of acyclovir into the body. Most people absorb only 15% to 20% of acyclovir, but the prodrug may boost absorption to the 50% to 80% range. In theory, valacyclovir should benefit patients who may not respond well to acyclovir because they aren't absorbing enough of the drug. It also has the advantage of less frequent dosing.

The second new prodrug is called famciclovir (brand name Famvir®). Developed by SmithKline Beecham, famciclovir is well absorbed by the body and then converts to penciclovir, the active ingredient. Like acyclovir, penciclovir works by sabotaging viral DNA. Famciclovir also appears to have an impressive "half-life," the length of time it remains active in the body. Like valacyclovir, famciclovir can be taken less often than acyclovir. Also like acyclovir, penciclovir is available in a cream formulation (brand name

Denavir®). However, this cream has not been studied for genital herpes, and its effectiveness is unknown.

FIRST EPISODES

Oral antiviral medication is commonly used for patients having a first episode. Here, given the large amounts of HSV present, and given the immune system's lack of experience in fighting the virus, medication can have dramatic results.

Taken for 7 to 10 days, antiviral medication can shorten the duration of herpes symptoms (itching and pain, for instance) by 40% to 50%. It can reduce the length of time during which a first-episode patient is "shedding virus"—in other words, contagious—by 70% to 80%. And overall, it can mean a 30% to 40% decrease in the total time it takes for skin to heal. Not everyone has a painful first episode, but if you're suffering through one, these statistics may spell welcome relief. Recommended dosages for a first episode are acyclovir 400 mg three times a day, acyclovir 200 mg five times a day, famciclovir 250 mg three times a day, or valacyclovir 1,000 mg (1 gram) twice a day.

RECURRENT EPISODES

Does antiviral therapy work against recurrent genital herpes too? It can, and here patients face a choice between two kinds of treatment. The first, called "episodic therapy," means using medication to halt or shorten an outbreak once it has started. The second option, called "suppressive therapy," means taking medicine every day in the hope that this will short-circuit reactivations of HSV and prevent outbreaks from occurring.

EPISODIC THERAPY: In this approach, a patient begins taking medication at the first sign of prodrome and continues for five days. (It's called "episodic" because one treats the individual episode and then stops taking medication until the next outbreak.) The results of episodic therapy vary quite a bit from person to person, but large controlled trials suggest the average: Episodic oral therapy generally reduces the time to healing by one to two days. If taken at the first sign of prodrome, in some cases episodic therapy can prevent an outbreak from occurring. Viral shedding, the period of contagiousness, may be reduced by up to 50%. Duration of symptoms (pain, tenderness, itching, tingling) may be reduced by 15% to 20%.

Recommended dosages are: acyclovir 400 mg three times a day, acyclovir 200 mg five times a day, acyclovir 800 mg twice a day, famciclovir 125 mg twice a day, or valacyclovir 500 mg twice a day.

As you can see from the discussion above, antiviral therapy used for recurrent genital herpes gives less dramatic results than it does in first episodes. This is partly explained by the fact that the immune system is doing a lot of the work already. That's why recurrent outbreaks are usually much shorter than first episodes, anyway. Many people feel the additional gains from episodic therapy are marginal, but for others medication offers a useful way to manage outbreaks.

Episodic therapy has its best results when medication is begun at the first sign of prodrome. For this reason, those taking episodic therapy should keep a supply of medication on hand so that they can self-initiate treatment when they first notice prodromal symptoms. The time required to involve a health-care provider in this decision and obtain medication causes a significant delay in the start of treatment and is impractical. Most health-care providers, therefore, will be open to this arrangement. The reality is that if recurrent lesions are already present, therapy offers little benefit.

SUPPRESSIVE THERAPY: Some people have outbreaks that are frequent or especially troublesome. In this case, one option is "suppressive therapy." This means taking antiviral medication every day to hold HSV in check, so that it's less likely to flare up and cause symptoms. Daily suppressive therapy reduces the number of outbreaks by at least 75% among people with frequent recurrences (that is, six or more outbreaks a year). For some people, suppressive therapy can prevent outbreaks altogether. Recommended dosages are: acyclovir 400 mg twice a day, famciclovir 250 mg twice a day, or valacyclovir which can be taken 500 mg once a day, 1,000 mg once a day, or 250 mg twice a day. The latter two regimens are recommended for persons with very frequent recurrences (10 or more a year).

As in the case of Teri, at the start of this chapter, many people find that suppressive antiviral treatment radically changes their experience of herpes, especially if they have frequent outbreaks. A number of long-term studies have enrolled people who had frequent recurrences, put them on an acyclovir dose of 400 mg twice daily, and carefully tracked the results. After five years, researchers have reported that nearly all patients on suppressive therapy have a dramatic reduction in the number of their outbreaks, beginning in the first year. They've also found that people on this regimen actually experience fewer and fewer recurrences as time goes on, so that after one year more than half of patients on suppressive therapy were completely free of outbreaks in any given year. A total of 20% of study participants had no outbreaks for the entire five years of the study. Famciclovir and valacyclovir, both approved in 1995, have fewer years of history behind them, but short-term studies have shown that both can also dramatically reduce the number of outbreaks for most people.

While suppressive therapy can be remarkably successful, it's important to note that some individuals simply do not respond this well to antiviral medication. In some cases, an increased dose is required to suppress HSV. For example, those who do not respond well to acyclovir may need as much as 800 mg twice daily. In fewer cases still, antivirals just aren't effective, suggesting the need for a different approach.

On the other end of the spectrum, people sometimes experiment with taking a smaller dose of antivirals, reporting that they need only 400 mg per day of acyclovir instead of the usual 800 mg, for example. It isn't wise, however, to experiment with dosages very much. Various regimens have been studied, and it's clear that for most people, one of the recommended dosages is the best choice. Taking too little increases the risk of breakthrough outbreaks, both symptomatic and subclinical. And taking more than is recommended may be a waste of money. If you want to alter the recommended suppressive therapy regimen, it's a good idea to discuss the issue with your medical professional.

Those on suppressive therapy may wish to stay on the drug indefinitely. But many experts in the field argue that most patients should consider suspending suppressive treatment after 12 consecutive months for what amounts to a reality check. Sometimes they won't have any outbreaks even without the drug, probably because of HSV's tendency to become less active after a number of years. Some people also find that their recurrences are less bothersome, so that they no longer want to take daily medication. The problem is that you have no way of knowing unless treatment is stopped for a while. For patients who continue to have troublesome recurrences, therapy can be renewed.

SAFETY CONCERNS

Over the years, many people with herpes have written ASHA with questions about the long-term safety of antiviral medication, particularly as used in suppressive therapy. Do these drugs have any toxic effects? Is suppressive therapy likely to give rise to "drug-resistant" strains of the virus, or to weaken the body's natural immune response?

Suppressive therapy with acyclovir has been studied in thousands of patients over the past decade, and so far it appears to be very safe. In large trials, a small number of patients report side effects such as headaches, nausea, or diarrhea, but overall these complaints are rare. Researchers also have run laboratory tests to check for systemic effects of the drug on liver function, white blood cell counts, and various other indexes of good health. So far, there is no evidence it causes harm to any internal organs. This is true even for those who have been taking acyclovir continuously as part of a five-year study and a smaller group who has taken acyclovir for 10 years. It will be years before researchers have gathered as much data on valacyclovir and famciclovir as they have now on acyclovir. However, thus far the safety data on the newer drugs are comparable to those for acyclovir.

The issue of resistant strains is more complicated. Within the universe of type 2 herpes simplex, there are many different "strains" of the virus. For the most part, the differences among them are relevant only to molecular biologists. Some strains, however, actually lack the enzyme (called thymidine kinase) that triggers acyclovir and enables the drug to thwart the virus in its effort to spread. Acyclovir is not active against strains lacking this enzyme, and famciclovir and valacyclovir aren't either. However, the immune system can control these viral strains in healthy people without the help of antiviral drugs, partly because the strains that lack thymidine kinase may be somewhat crippled.

In patients who have weakened immune systems, however, these strains can cause serious illness, because the immune system can't do its customary work in suppressing herpes, and resistant strains can replicate without much interference. People with AIDS, for example, may have severe herpes outbreaks that do not heal on acyclovir. Alternate treatments are now being used for these patients.

Is the problem of drug resistance likely to increase over time, as more and more people take antivirals? This is a controversial issue, but it appears unlikely. On one hand, researchers have actually checked samples of HSV taken before the development of acyclovir, and they find a small percentage of viral strains that are naturally less sensitive to the drug. Given this finding, resistance would appear to be more a matter of chance or of immune deficiency than the result of acyclovir use. On the other hand, some

scientists believe that HSV does mutate over time, and it's possible that acyclovir—or any antiviral drug—will exert pressure for
certain strains of the virus to survive better than others.

For now, the experts say, the odds of developing acyclovir-
resistant herpes are extremely low in people with normal immune
systems; in fact, there has been only one documented case to date.
Researchers have looked for resistant strains in people who have
been taking acyclovir for a week, a year, or several years. So far,
they don't find evidence of increasing resistance in the general
population, though this will undoubtedly be a subject for further
study. The issue of drug-resistance in those with weakened
immunity, by contrast, is certainly a legitimate concern, and
immunocompromised patients with genital herpes should be
monitored closely if they're taking antiviral medication.

While some people worry about the safety of an antiviral
drug like acyclovir, others get so enthusiastic as to lose sight of
the facts. Suppressive acyclovir works well for many patients and
can actually get rid of herpes symptoms for a time, but it should
not be considered a "cure." Even with suppressive acyclovir, the
virus remains poised for a return to action.

ANTIVIRALS AND SUBCLINICAL SHEDDING

While antivirals can be successful in controlling herpes
symptoms, researchers only recently have turned their attention to
the important issue of antiviral therapy and subclinical shedding.
Does suppressive therapy lower the risk of unrecognized herpes
reactivation as well as curb recognized outbreaks? Does it change
the odds of spreading herpes to a sexual partner?

One study addressing this question found that women on suppressive acyclovir (400 mg, twice daily) experienced a 94% reduction in subclinical shedding while taking daily therapy. Another study found that women on various doses of suppressive famciclovir experienced an 80% to 90% reduction in subclinical shedding. Given that antivirals can reduce viral shedding both with symptoms and without, it's logical to suppose that treatment has an impact on transmission. The researchers who conducted these studies, however, caution that even daily therapy did not totally block viral shedding, and the amounts of virus isolated on some days of shedding were probably sufficient to cause transmission. Because of its obvious importance to people with herpes and to public health, the role of therapy as a means of preventing the spread of the infection should be examined closely. A study of whether suppressive valacyclovir can help prevent transmission is now under way.

COMPARISON SHOPPING

How does one evaluate the available treatments? Let's consider four major aspects: effectiveness, safety, convenience and cost.

In terms of effectiveness, clinical studies have not found any significant differences among acyclovir, famciclovir, and valacyclovir in terms of their effectiveness for people with established HSV infection. All three appear to work for the vast majority of patients as a suppressive therapy, and to have modest but predictable benefit as an episodic therapy.

As far as safety, it can be argued that acyclovir has an edge by virtue of its long track record, with no evidence of toxicity even in those who have been taking daily medication for years. However, the newer drugs also appear to be very safe and have few side effects. Valacyclovir, which uses acyclovir as its active ingredient, has shown a similar safety profile so far, as has famciclovir. Perhaps, with time, the prodrugs will match acyclovir's record fully.

Convenience probably offers an edge to the newer drugs. Valacyclovir and famciclovir can be taken twice daily as episodic therapies for recurrent herpes, as compared with three to five times daily for acyclovir. For suppression, valacyclovir achieves good results with a once-daily dose, something that neither of its competitors has been able to match.

In the end, however, cost may be the most dramatic variable. In the era of managed care, a given patient's therapeutic options are highly dependent on the insurer's regulations and policies. One type of health plan might place generic acyclovir in its formulary; another might go with one of the prodrugs. The release of acyclovir as a generic drug has brought a sharp drop in its price and may ultimately bring about adjustments in the prices of the newer medicines. Given the competitive nature of the marketplace, it would be wise for people considering a long-term course of therapy to research the cost of each of the three drugs to determine which is the best value. For suppressive therapy, for example, what is the cost to you of twice daily generic acyclovir versus once daily valacyclovir? In the end, all three antivirals can be considered safe and effective, but the hit to one's pocketbook may vary dramatically according to health insurance, geography, and the pricing structure at your preferred local pharmacy.

OTHER PRESCRIPTION MEDICATIONS

Acyclovir, famciclovir, and valacyclovir are likely to represent the "front line" in drug therapies for the majority of genital herpes patients. But there are some other antiviral medications in use for special situations.

Foscarnet is now in use as an alternative therapy for immuno-compromised patients who don't respond well to acyclovir. Like acyclovir, foscarnet is able to block viral replication, but it does so by working directly against a viral enzyme called polymerase. The drug has been helpful, particularly to people with AIDS, but it has several disadvantages. First, it isn't readily absorbed through the stomach, and must be administered intravenously. Second, it has many toxic side effects. It's not currently recommended for patients with normal immune function.

Another antiviral compound, trifluridine, is occasionally used to treat herpes infections that do not heal on acyclovir. Drug-makers also have tried to develop effective topical ointments or gels. Some, like topical acyclovir, work directly against the virus, but it's been difficult to make a drug that's absorbed through the skin well enough to provide effective relief from symptoms. Virostat®, a product now on the market in Canada, has made some limited claims of efficacy. Using the antiviral edoxudine as its active ingredient, Virostat® has been shown to reduce the time of viral shedding. The cream also appears to ease symptoms very slightly in women, while bringing no benefit to men.

Still other topical drugs make no claim to stop viral replication but may relieve symptoms in other ways. One of these is topical lidocaine, which partially (and temporarily) numbs the nerve endings and is occasionally used in primary episodes. It's not widely used for herpes, and people using it should be aware of the possibility of allergic reactions to this and similar drugs such as novocaine.

Other topical medications, too—even prescription drugs—have their down side when it comes to herpes. Some doctors use topical steroid creams to reduce inflammation and speed healing for a variety of skin problems. Unfortunately, steroids cause some immune impairment, and this may make matters worse, decreasing the ability of the skin to heal on its own. Steroids are not effective for HSV, and they can prolong herpes outbreaks. Topical steroids may increase the risk of yeast infection as well. (By the way, people taking steroids for other conditions, such as asthma, sometimes report that their herpes outbreaks are worse as a result.)

OVER-THE-COUNTER MEDICATIONS

In ASHA's 1991 survey, most patients had tried between two and five different therapies for genital herpes. Some of these were not strictly drugs but dietary supplements or nutritional approaches. Some were various types of stress reduction or psychotherapy. These strategies are discussed in Chapter Thirteen.

Most of the medications for genital herpes fall under the previous sections on antivirals, but there are a few others worth noting. In particular, people with herpes sometimes try over-the-counter products to relieve symptoms when they have flare-ups. It's difficult to assess the value of these medications because they generally are not tested as rigorously as the other drugs covered here. As such, they are not evaluated in the scientific literature.

In some cases, they are not labeled specifically for use in the treatment of genital herpes, either. They nonetheless attract attention through word-of-mouth, or because they claim to erase whatever kind of symptom is most distressing to the patient—itching, for example.

Unfortunately, topical creams may actually delay the healing of herpes outbreaks. In some cases, the creams contain alcohol compounds that might dry the skin to the point where it is easily chafed. Other topical treatments, such as Campho-Phenique®, may make patients feel better because the product contains phenol. Like xylocaine, and like the lidocaine mentioned earlier, phenol numbs the area locally, without treating the actual infection. Some people may find this useful. It's important to note, however, that products such as Campho-Phenique® or Blistex® do not actually work directly against the virus—they concentrate instead on the symptoms of viral attack.

If you want more information about a prescription or over-the-counter product for treating symptoms of genital herpes, one option is to contact the Office of Consumer Affairs in the FDA. (See the Resource List on page 195.) They can discuss drugs that are labeled specifically for treatment of genital herpes. Another option is to contact the product's manufacturer.

CONSIDERING TREATMENT FOR YOURSELF

Is antiviral therapy something to consider for yourself? There are no simple guidelines to offer, because every patient is affected by variables that are unique to his or her situation. These center on the patient's medical history and attitude toward medications, and on the health-care provider's views regarding treatment. Talking with your medical professional about the various treatment options may be useful. Here are some issues to weigh:

• Do you really want medication? Antiviral drugs are extremely helpful for some people in regaining a feeling of control over their lives. Most people with herpes, however, don't feel the need to take medication, because their outbreaks are relatively mild. And some just don't like the idea of taking medication if they don't really have to.

• Are outbreaks painful? A majority of respondents in the 1991 ASHA survey rate the pain of recurrent outbreaks as "minimal" or "moderate," but some patients have severe pain and discomfort. Your doctor has no way to gauge this other than your honest assessment. Try to communicate this information.

• Are you having outbreaks often? A pattern of recurrent outbreaks six or more times a year leads some patients to use suppressive antiviral therapy, especially if the outbreaks are lengthy or painful. But the threshold is different for everyone. In any case, your doctor will probably want to know what your pattern is. It may be a good idea to keep track if you're interested in suppressive antiviral treatment.

• Does recurrent herpes take an emotional toll on you? Even people who get just a handful of outbreaks each year may feel the need for therapy if, for example, they are facing a time of stress during which herpes is the "last thing" they want to contend with. One example: Persons recently divorced or on their own after the breakup of a long-term relationship might suddenly feel anxiety about herpes and seek advice on treatment for the first time.

• Can you afford the medication? Antiviral therapies can be costly. Suppressive regimens, for example, can cost dollars per day. Some patients are covered for costs of medication under their health insurance policies.

• Are you pregnant, or trying to get pregnant? Most of the medications mentioned here should not be used during pregnancy, except in very specific circumstances. (See Chapter Fourteen for more on herpes in pregnancy.)

• Are you and your partner very concerned about the risk of transmission? The usefulness of antiviral medication in helping prevent transmission has not been proven, but for people who want to do everything they can to reduce the risk, suppressive therapy can be a reasonable addition to other prevention strategies.

9

TAKING CONTROL:
THE EMOTIONAL ISSUES

*"When I acquired herpes seven months ago," says Sean, "I was
shattered. I remember sitting there in the dark listening to Pink Floyd's
'Comfortably Numb,' which is exactly what I was (thanks to the sedatives
my doctor had given me)."*

Not everyone finds herpes a major challenge emotionally, but
many people do—especially at the beginning. It can change your
self-image in profound ways, threaten intimate relationships, and
lead you to withdraw from close friends as well.

In ASHA's 1991 survey, signs of emotional stress were quite
common during the period following a first episode. These
included feelings of depression, noted by 82% of respondents,
fear of rejection (75%), feelings of isolation (69%), fear of dis-
covery (55%), and self-destructive feelings (27%).

Many of those surveyed, however, had been coping with herpes for several years. Interestingly, when they were asked about
the most recent 12 months (prior to the survey), the results were
markedly different: Fewer people had the same fears and feelings.

It's clear from the survey and from contact with many other
herpes patients that the time immediately following a herpes

diagnosis is the hardest. For some it presents a number of personal challenges that have more to do with psychology than medicine. And patients often meet these by going through several stages of adjustment.

HERPES AND SELF-IMAGE

Alexandra got herpes when she was still in her teens, and she says the experience caused her to question her own worth over and over again. "I had times," she writes, "when I would feel very unattractive and feel like I was different from everyone my own age. The best way I can sum it up is that I felt 'dirty.'"

Why does herpes have the power to alter our self-image? In some ways this is truly a paradox. HSV is a common virus, and certainly most adults already carry HSV-1 anyway. Most of us have had other herpesviruses as well. It's true that genital herpes has the potential to recur more frequently than the other herpesviruses. But this alone doesn't seem worth all the strain and upheaval. In the end, genital herpes is burdensome because it raises issues of sexuality. And in our society that brings with it a load of emotional baggage.

Some of the problems begin with society and the most basic attitudes we develop about sexual activity. Many of us grow up without a clear sense that the sexual drive is a normal part of being human. Instead, it's characterized as dirty, hidden in the shadows. We're often taught that it's something you don't discuss in public. In fact, going back to the turn of the century, this polite silence is one of the reasons that sexually transmitted diseases (such as syphilis) spread unchecked, with few efforts made to prevent them or find better treatments. Social reformers decried what they called a "conspiracy of silence" that enabled the continued spread of these venereal diseases.

Today, we're surrounded by the imagery of sex in our arts and entertainment industries and in the marketing of products as diverse as soft drinks and automobiles. Yet the prevailing message at the personal level is little changed. At best, we have no consensus about such a thing as a "healthy sex life," and many would argue that our society has no concept of this at all. As a result, we can't talk openly about aspects of sex such as disease prevention. You see a lot of sexual innuendo on television, for example, but a public service message advocating the use of condoms for safe sex can still touch off a raging debate.

One consequence is that diseases spread through sexual contact take on added complications. People come to feel that having an STD is much more than a medical problem. Instead it becomes something for which you suffer not only symptoms but shame. A part of the reason that a mundane illness like HSV would cause depression or social withdrawal is that we blame ourselves and fear the blame that may be placed on us by others. Many people like Alexandra feel branded or implicitly accused of having done something wrong.

People also lose perspective about the medical implications of herpes. Too often we see health as an all-or-nothing proposition—we are either healthy or unhealthy, with no middle ground. And some people regard a chronic infection like herpes as the end of health. We become somehow "imperfect."

In reality, however, health involves a process of growth and change. Everyone faces a host of physical challenges as inevitable as life itself. The task is to meet them head on and get past them. Herpesviruses are no exception. One gets "mono," waits out the period of illness, and then moves on. In the end, we should consider ourselves healthy because we meet the challenges that life throws our way.

The message, above all, is that we must believe in our competence—our ability to handle the challenges posed by all sorts of infections. In order to do this we must keep things in perspective. We must frame a problem like herpes as a reality that requires some adjustments, but refuse to let it change our view of ourselves.

HERPES AND RELATIONSHIPS

In the end, of course, it's very difficult to separate the issues of self-image from the worries people have about the practical impact of herpes on important relationships. Will close friends shun you? Do you dare tell them? Will herpes destroy a sexual relationship you have now? Will a future romantic interest understand and accept the news? Will you be able to remain sexually active?

Perhaps the most pressing worry for those newly diagnosed with herpes is the reaction of a sexual partner. Patients often say they fear telling a partner or a romantic interest because they're afraid of being rejected. "I've had herpes for three months now, and I've been avoiding any sexual entanglements," writes Pat. "I'm not ready to tell anyone. I just don't think I'll be able to handle it if someone dumps me because of this. And I imagine there's a good chance of that."

These fears are natural. But they're also apt to grow enormously out of proportion to the problem. Firstly, it's not unusual for people with herpes to go through a phase of doubting their attractiveness or desirability without having any basis for doing so. If you find you're doubting yourself in this way, remind yourself that herpes is essentially invisible, except when you're having an outbreak. (And even then it's usually visible only to you.) Secondly, if it's unbearable to think that you may not always be able to have sex when you want, consider that there is a good chance you'll face other interruptions in your sex life as well. What about the pressures of work, travel, family emergencies, pregnancy and childbirth, or a variety of illnesses? The point is, no one is sexually available all the time.

What about rejection? This does happen, and in the two surveys conducted by ASHA 20% to 25% of respondents reported at least one instance of being rejected by a partner because of herpes.

Every year, we get calls and letters from people who share details of how a disclosure about herpes has caused upheaval—a promising romance that sputters, for example, or a long-standing relationship that ends. But it's interesting to note how often people close these letters with words of hope or optimism. Typical is a letter from Sara, whose boyfriend had infected her unwittingly and then made matters worse by saying, "Maybe now you won't leave me." Sara left this man and dated cautiously for a while before "finding a gem," Bruce. "I dated Bruce for over two months before I had the courage to tell him," she writes. "The night I told him, he went back to his place for clothes (for work the next day) and spent the night with me. Since then, he's been patient with my outbreaks and psychological fears, and we've been a happy loving couple for over a year now."

For Sara, as for many others, the pain of rejection becomes a path to finding someone more mature and more loving.

When struggling to adjust to having herpes, it's natural to conjure up some of the worst-case scenarios. And certainly there are stories and jokes about herpes that fuel this kind of anxiety.

Sadly, much less is said about the thousands of real-life stories, like Sara's, that contradict the "bad press." You're likely to find a wealth of them in a local herpes support group, where members typically spend a good deal of time talking about the fear of rejection and the experiences people have when they're searching for a loving companion.

ASHA also has interviewed many couples about this issue and found no indication that herpes has to stand in the way of successful, enduring relationships. One woman who doesn't have herpes wrote ASHA with the specific aim of making this very point. "So many people with herpes seem to give up on relationships," she commented, "so I wanted to share my story. My husband is the love of my life. We've been married almost 10 years, and herpes hasn't spoiled our relationship in any way. Like almost everyone else, we've had our problems, but herpes isn't one of them."

Asked about herpes and long-term relationships, psychologists concur that HSV is basically a non-issue in a healthy relationship. As long as two people are honest with each other at the start, as long as they can talk about herpes and make choices about it, the infection itself becomes just one more practical matter to deal with—usually a small one. If herpes triggers a lot of tension in a relationship, the experts say, often there are some underlying problems.

Of course, it's not always easy to get over the initial hurdles. Talking about herpes, even with someone you love and trust, can be daunting at first. And being sexually intimate with someone means having to discuss the risk of spreading herpes. This brings with it the need for some choices about prevention—choices that, ideally, you will make as a couple. Telling a partner and thinking through the issue of prevention are explored in depth in the next two chapters.

As for the wider social circle, herpes is not nearly as big an issue, but it can present a dilemma. With time, the vast majority of people learn to talk with doctors, with friends, and certainly with lovers. But there are those who fall into a kind of social paralysis. Perhaps they find herpes such a painful subject that they can't bring themselves to talk to a doctor about it. Perhaps they've been diagnosed with herpes and can't find it within themselves to tell the person they're dating. Some people break off intimate relationships rather than admit having herpes. And this kind of withdrawal can lead to a more general isolation. People caught in this bind let herpes become the defining reality in their lives.

This behavior sometimes can result in a syndrome of "self-fulfilling prophecy." Feeling isolated, people may look around and conclude that others have withdrawn from them. In reality, the isolation is their own doing, but the tendency is to blame others—to assume that people no longer like them as much because of herpes.

Psychologist Cal VanderPlate, who has studied the behavioral effects of herpes, says that the key to keeping herpes in perspective is communication. People who can tell a lover or a friend about herpes often get emotional support from this person when they need it. If they're worried about having an outbreak, for example, they can talk about it. And this emotional support is crucial. It reduces the anxiety a person may feel about having herpes, and it may possibly lessen the number of stress-related outbreaks a person will have over time. VanderPlate says this kind of "herpes-specific support" usually comes from a spouse or lover, but it can come from a friend as well. In any case, the key is having someone to talk to, but this requires honesty and openness on the part of the person with herpes. Usually, says VanderPlate, acceptance and support are just around the corner, but we never know unless we take the risk.

This doesn't mean, of course, that *everyone* has to know about herpes. Your health is a private matter, and herpes affects only a small part of life anyway. While privacy is reasonable, though, experts warn that absolute *secrecy* can be a sign of trouble, because it requires an ever-watchful state of mind to maintain the secret, and can encourage a tendency toward social paralysis.

WHAT YOU CAN DO

- Realize that it's normal to be stressed emotionally by herpes, especially at first. Give yourself some time to adjust, and remember that the emotional issues will get easier.

• Pick one close friend you can talk to about herpes and tell him or her about it. You can ask that the conversation be kept in absolute confidence.

• If you've had herpes for several months or more, assess your progress in adjusting to it. Are you angry? Have you withdrawn socially? Do you completely avoid sexual relationships? Can you talk about herpes? If you're still extremely angry about having herpes or are unable to talk about it with anyone, keep in mind that this may be an indication of trouble. Giving up on sexual relationships might be one also.

• Everyone is different, and it may just take more time before you feel you've got your life back where you want it. But it might also be that something is blocking your way forward. If things aren't getting easier with time, you may need a helping hand. Many people seek advice from a health-care provider, counselor or psychotherapist; others may prefer a support group. Consider whether there is something you can do that would help you to take control again and get on with your life. Above all, don't give up on yourself, and don't assume you're doomed to a life of loneliness. You're not.

• Some people resume dating but worry that herpes will prevent them from having successful long-term relationships. The news media are not exactly full of herpes "success stories," but this is no reason to despair. With more than 40 million adults carrying HSV-2, herpes becomes just a minor issue in countless relationships. These stand or fall on far more important issues. Erase the idea that HSV will undermine your ability to have successful relationships.

10

TELLING YOUR PARTNER

Carl, now 38, remembers the first few conversations he had about herpes. "When I got the diagnosis I was able to make phone calls to the two people I'd slept with and ask if either of them had any idea they had herpes. But later, when it came time to tell someone new, I lost my nerve at first. I really couldn't stand the idea that it might make someone feel differently about me."

The prospect of telling another person you have herpes can cause you to worry, and the stakes are often highest when you're getting ready to tell someone with whom you'd like to be sexually intimate. What will this person say? Laugh? Cry? Walk out on you? Accept that herpes doesn't have to be a big deal?

The outcome of this conversation is not completely in your control. But there are things you can do to shape the message and the response. And if you're planning on having sex with anybody—herpes or no herpes—it's important to realize that both parties have a right to an honest discussion about possible risks. There are many sexually transmitted infections, some of them much more damaging than herpes. So *you* have something to gain from knowing your potential partner's sexual history, too.

MAKING THE CHOICE

As some people ponder having this kind of "heart-to-heart" with a lover or romantic interest, they begin to wonder if it's really necessary. Why risk rejection, they reason, when there may be another way? What about just avoiding sex during herpes outbreaks, and practicing safer sex in between?

Certainly there are individuals who choose not to tell a sex partner about herpes or who find it impossible to tell until *after* they've had sex. There are countless combinations of people and circumstances, and no book such as this can presume to anticipate them all. In couples who pursue an ongoing relationship, however, it can be quite helpful if herpes isn't a secret locked away from your lover.

For one thing, the secrecy itself is likely to cause more anxiety than telling the truth. The closer you become, the more you'll want to be honest—yet the task at hand is likely to get harder over time. If and when you do finally disclose the truth, suddenly there are two issues on the table. One is herpes. But potentially more explosive is the issue of trust.

Withholding the truth has other disadvantages as well. It puts the entire burden of preventing the spread of herpes on one person, and it may force the invention of lies and half-truths to postpone sexual activity during outbreaks. These phony excuses may in themselves undermine a relationship, and they place an additional psychological stress on the person who's keeping a secret. There also are ethical and legal implications. Everyone has the right to make an informed choice about his or her sexual partner, and the courts have ruled in some cases that failure to disclose a sexually transmitted infection like herpes may be grounds for a lawsuit. (These suits aren't common, but some individuals do choose to bring legal action. See Chapter Nineteen for further discussion.)

It's clear that keeping herpes a secret from your lover can fuel emotional stress, but there are health-related issues at stake as well. Just as your partner may be at risk for herpes, he or she may place you at risk for a number of other STDs. Chlamydia, genital warts, gonorrhea, trichomoniasis—all these are sexually transmitted, and all of them cause more new infections each year than herpes does. Some also have more serious consequences. And of course there is the risk of acquiring human immunodeficiency virus (HIV), the cause of AIDS. So it makes sense to talk about herpes in the context of overall sexual health. This approach equalizes people from the beginning and can help to preserve self-esteem on both sides.

In reality, questions about risks to your health are relevant to both partners: Have you had another lover in the past? Have you used condoms? Have you ever had a sexually transmitted disease? Do you realize that you can have HIV or other STDs and not know it? These may be difficult issues to raise, but frank discussion about these things is becoming the norm in more relationships all the time.

Honesty and open communication not only pave the way for making smart choices about prevention, they also carry emotional benefits, not the least of which are mutual trust and respect. Sometimes the person who is newly diagnosed feels reluctant to tell anyone about herpes. But psychologists have found that telling a sexual partner is very important in making the adjustment to herpes and learning to cope with it. Herpes or no herpes, communication and sharing are two of the cornerstones for any successful relationship. What's more, behavioral research has shown that the most effective emotional support for people with herpes comes from their lovers or close friends.

STARTING WITH YOURSELF

Once you've decided to tell a partner about herpes, it may prove helpful to think through the process and anticipate some of the potential issues.

First, it's important to consider whether you've come to terms with herpes yourself and accepted that it's not such an earth-shaking problem. There is little to gain from opening up to others about herpes if you're likely to characterize it in the most negative way or if you are still punishing yourself over it.

Many health-care professionals with experience in this area believe that self-esteem is a crucial element in coping with herpes. Some argue that self-esteem may require specific work, in which you attempt to replace negative attitudes toward yourself with positive ones. If herpes has radically altered the way you see yourself, you may benefit from actually thinking through and writing down these issues or getting feedback from a trusted friend, a counselor, or a herpes support group. (See the Resource List, page 195.)

Whether or not you find it necessary to assess your self-esteem in this way, it's a good idea to know the key facts about herpes and feel comfortable in discussing them. Be prepared for a range of questions—some of them thought-provoking and some of them banal. Remember: Myths and misinformation about herpes are commonplace. You probably know a great deal by now, but you have to assume that your audience is starting from scratch. Some of the points you might want to highlight include the following:

• HSV is the same virus that causes cold sores on the lips and face. Just as herpes can flare up from time to time on the face, it also can cause genital sores every so often.

• Most people carry either HSV-1 or HSV-2, and about one in four adults has genital herpes. It's usually so mild, however, that many people don't know they have it.

• Herpes can be spread during sexual contact when sores or other symptoms are present, and there may be a risk of transmission at other times.

• Herpes is frequently spread by people who don't know they're infected. Since they haven't been diagnosed, they don't recognize their symptoms as being contagious. Even people who have received a "clean bill of health" from a doctor or STD clinic may have undiagnosed genital herpes, since most standard blood tests are unreliable for detecting HSV-2.

• Once diagnosed, a person can take precautions to lower the risk of spreading herpes.

Some people also like to have brochures or other educational materials on hand when they talk about herpes. These may give you added credibility, and your partner may want to do some reading on his or her own. You have everything to gain from helping to promote this process. You can also give a partner the telephone number of the National Herpes Hotline. (See the Resource List, page 195.)

Having a partner take matters under advisement or go elsewhere for information isn't easy, but it's reasonable to expect that someone who is new to the idea of herpes will need time to absorb the facts and check their own feelings. And the outcome can be very satisfying, as in the case of Lauren. "I contracted herpes five years ago from a partner who failed to tell me that he had it," she writes. "I have slowly come to terms with my anger towards him and myself. Since that time, I have been sexually active with several men. Each time, I chose to tell them about herpes *before* getting sexually involved. In every case, they eventually agreed that herpes should not get in the way of our sex life. Sometimes they needed time or needed to read some literature before making a decision, and one man even consulted his doctor. My point is simply that if you give a person the choice to understand what herpes is about, and you practice safer sex, you can have an active social and sexual life."

PREPARING TO TELL: WHEN AND HOW

Above all, the suggestions offered here are just ways to make it easier for you to think through the task of telling a partner. Each person will have a style and presentation that's unique, and no one should feel constrained to use a schedule or a script that just doesn't fit the situation. However you proceed, though, your attitude and your mood will have a great deal of influence on how the news is received. People tend to behave the way you expect them to behave, and a gloomy presentation may well increase the chance of a gloomy response. So the key is: Be positive and be confident. Expect that your partner will be accepting and supportive. You are doing the right thing for both of you.

When is the best time? People who have shared their experiences through herpes support groups or ASHA's newsletters tend to agree that it's usually best to allow a relationship to develop a bit before bringing up the subject. There is sometimes pressure to become sexually involved early in a relationship. But in the current era of HIV and so many other STDs, it's safest to pursue a policy of moving slowly. In this view, you wait until the time is right for a talk about sexual histories on both sides.

A partner may become impatient, but if there is real affection between you, he or she will wait it out and will understand that you respect yourself. This in turn will bring home the message that you're a safer partner than those who are willing to take the plunge with zero information. If pressured, for example, you might say: "I really like you, and I'm getting comfortable with you, but I'd rather hold off on sex for now. I really want to trust you and know you before we have sex."

If you do become interested in someone and begin to feel comfortable in the relationship, you can prepare yourself and look for logical opportunities to broach the subject. A television or newspaper report on AIDS, for instance, might naturally start a conversation about safer sex.

of the fact that you want a dialogue, so it's best not to go on at great length. You're wanting a discussion, not a lecture or confession.

Once the words are out, it's a good idea to ask your partner some questions to elicit his or her thoughts. You might say, for example, "Do you know anything about herpes?" Or, "Do you know anyone who gets cold sores?"

Sometimes the initial reaction may be one of confusion, distress, or silence. There is always the possibility that a partner will be upset initially, though in many cases the person simply needs time to sort things out. You might try a technique like "active listening" and say something like: "You seem to be getting upset about all of this. Tell me what you're thinking, or feeling. Maybe I can answer your questions."

Clearly, if there are countless approaches, there are an equal number of subtleties in the responses you might get. Some people may overreact, some won't bat an eye. Given the number of people who have herpes, many will have had this discussion before. Whatever the reaction, try to be flexible yourself. Remember that it took you time to adjust as well, and that the first response is not always the one that counts.

At the same time, some experts say, don't be overly concerned about protecting the feelings of your partner. You want him or her to have the time needed to process this information, yes. But after all, you have needs yourself. And you probably don't need a relationship in which you have to do all the emotional work. Will your partner be there for you when you need someone? Has he or she made you feel safe? It's important to assess the other person's behavior when presented with the challenge of a safer sex discussion. People who are judgmental, those who have a very narrow life experience, or those who are excessively afraid of germs may not be good candidates for your love.

It's natural for people with herpes to worry about rejection—especially at first. But many people write to ASHA with a very different perspective after they've had a chance to reflect on their experiences. An instance of rejection can also be seen as "quality control," as in the case of a San Francisco couple who shared their story in a letter. "My wife and I each contracted genital herpes before we met," the man recounts. "We went through difficult times and relationships, but these made us emotionally stronger, and hopefully better people. Because each of us had been the victim of people who were dishonest, we had both decided to be honest with potential partners.

"We met after having lived with herpes independently for over three years. Before we became physically intimate, I disclosed to her that I had herpes. To my total surprise, she responded with the same statement. We were married nine months after our first meeting."

The safer sex discussion may help you to separate the wheat from the chaff. And it's generally accepted that it's best to find out early. It takes a lot more than the occasional aggravation of herpes to destroy a sound relationship. The bottom line is that there are lots of people out there who will be attracted to you for exactly who you are—with or without herpes.

The majority of people will react well. After all, you trust them enough to share a confidence with them that you probably wouldn't share with just anybody. Most people respect that. And in talking about safer sex, you've shown maturity in facing up to a

It's likely that herpes will bring some changes to your sex life, especially at first. But remember: it *does not* mean the end of sexuality. There are millions of other people who have genital herpes, and millions of couples who deal with it as little more than a minor inconvenience. You can make the adjustment, too. It may mean you'll have to be a bit more careful in some respects. But it does not have to be a heavy burden to bear throughout your life.

A lot of the choices you face hinge on the specifics of your personal situation. For example: What's your sexual orientation? Are you single? Are you in a long-term relationship? Do you have several sexual partners or just one? What are your sexual habits? Do you already practice safer sex? Do you have frequent outbreaks? All of the issues surrounding safer sex are very personal, posing decisions best made with your partner.

The desire to protect a sexual partner and prevent the spread of herpes is often very strong. The vast majority of people surveyed by ASHA lists this as one of their primary concerns. But as we've noted in Chapter Ten, there is another equally pressing side to the story. That's *your* health, and the need to protect yourself from other, potentially more serious sexually transmitted infections. As we've said, there are 12 million new sexually transmitted infections each year, and some experts say that 50% of adults—whatever their race, sex, or social class—will be infected with an STD at some point. With HIV/AIDS on the list, taking risks with sex can literally mean taking risks with your life. And many of these infections can remain hidden, so that those who carry them don't know about it.

The point is that sexual relationships are a two-way street.

You're aware that you carry HSV and are probably concerned to protect your partner from infection. But your current or future partner may carry an infection that could affect *your* health as well. It's very hard to know. In any case, you might begin to see reducing risk in sexual encounters as something that's in *your interest* as much as your partner's.

THE BASICS

First we'll focus on herpes by itself. Forget about whether you're gay or straight, coupled or single; forget about the other STDs. In the absence of all other factors, what you can do to prevent the spread of herpes boils down to two steps: (1) avoiding direct skin-to-skin contact with herpes lesions during obvious flare-ups; and (2) using condoms or taking other precautions between outbreaks as a guard against unrecognized herpes—the subclinical shedding discussed in Chapter Four. Both of these issues center on times when HSV has *reactivated*. The period during which you're actually contagious may in fact be a relatively small percentage of the time. Because it's unpredictable, however, the precautions needed to protect a partner deserve a detailed discussion.

During Outbreaks

The risk of spreading herpes is highest whenever symptoms, ranging from subtle to painful, are present. The tingling or itch of prodrome, for example, is a signal that virus has probably found its way to the skin and that there is risk of spreading HSV to a sexual partner. An itchy red patch of skin near the genitals

you may have virus on the skin or mucous membranes on 6% to 10% of days. Afterwards, you probably have subclinical shedding about 2% to 4% of the time, something on the order of two weeks out of the year. The problem is, you don't know which days these will be.

What can you do about it? For straight or gay couples practicing vaginal or anal intercourse, experts say that the most thorough approach is to use condoms between outbreaks. You recall that condoms were *not* recommended as protection *during* outbreaks, but they're considered a better bet for subclinical reactivation. It's complicated logic, but the reasoning goes like this:

Shedding can occur anywhere in the genital area, because HSV can travel any of the nerve pathways linked to the ganglion at the base of the spine. So condoms still aren't a complete guarantee, for instance, if you are shedding virus from the scrotum. The research to date, however, suggests that the biggest risk of transmission occurs when there is contact with surfaces such as the penis or the soft mucosal tissue of the vagina, cervix, or anus. For this reason, researchers say that condoms are indeed useful protection between outbreaks. In fact, one of the few studies in which men were tested daily found that the majority of subclinical shedding in males did occur on the penis, which means that condoms should help men with herpes protect their partners.

Another potential approach to lowering the risk of transmission during an unrecognized reactivation is to use suppressive therapy. While no one has proven that use of daily antivirals prevents transmission, they have been shown to reduce subclinical shedding by 80% to 94%, and further studies to see if antivirals reduce the risk of transmission are under way. Based on this, it seems probable that a combination of condom use and suppressive therapy would provide a high level of protection.

RISK REDUCTION FOR GAYS AND LESBIANS

The little data that have been gathered about the transmission of herpes stem primarily from research on heterosexual couples, but gays and lesbians often raise questions about the particular risks they may face. In addition, many people—both straight and gay—are eager to learn whether anything is known about the relative risks of various sexual acts.

Unfortunately, medical science has little to say about the probability of transmission through oral sex versus anal versus other types of sexual pleasuring. But there are some insights about herpes that may be particularly pertinent for gays and for lesbians.

Given the enormous impact of AIDS, people in the gay community are better informed about HIV prevention than most other segments of the U.S. population. The importance of herpes and other STDs as risk factors for acquiring HIV, however, has not always been well publicized. Specifically, research has shown that genital herpes—and, in fact, a number of other STDs—create tiny breaks in the skin and in mucosal tissue that give HIV a portal of entry. In addition, herpes lesions attract larger than average numbers of T-cells—precisely the kind of lymphocyte that HIV likes to attack. Given these two factors, the person who is experiencing a herpes outbreak or an episode of subclinical shedding has an especially high risk of getting infected with HIV *if* he or she is exposed to HIV. The "if" here is important, because it is *not true* that herpes puts one on some inevitable path to HIV. But the added risk of HIV is worth considering. For similar reasons, those who are HIV-positive and also have genital herpes are likely more efficient *transmitters* of HIV as well.

All of the above argues for the same kinds of precautions outlined previously, such as abstaining from sex during outbreaks and condom use at other times. Condoms have been studied more thoroughly for their efficacy in vaginal sex, but for over a decade the Centers for Disease Control has been recommending their use for anal and oral sex as well. For anal sex, water-based lubricants will likely offer an extra measure of protection, decreasing the likelihood of condom breakage and of trauma to the rectum that can result from anal intercourse.

In contrast to the situation with gay men, lesbians have been regarded as *unlikely* to acquire STDs such as herpes and HIV. And while the rates of some STDs are indeed lower in lesbians, a recent study at the University of Washington showed that some 13% of lesbian women tested positive for HSV-2. How do they acquire it? First, researchers point out that as many as 90% of women who identify themselves as lesbian have had sex with men at some point in their lives. Second, given the importance of oral sex in lesbian couples, it's likely that HSV is sometimes spread through oral-genital contact, and likely as well that there is a fairly high percentage of HSV-1 in lesbian women that represents latent genital infection. Third, it appears that women who have sex with women are able to transmit STDs such as genital HPV—and possibly herpes—through sex toys and through use of the hands for pleasuring.

In terms of prevention, researchers stress that women who have sex with women should be aware that oral sex does pose a risk of transmission. In this regard, some women use household plastic wrap as a safer sex barrier during cunnilingus, and some use nonpowdered latex gloves, which can be cut to a suitable flat shape for oral sex. As far as for sex toys, it's important to understand that viruses or bacteria deposited on the toy by one person can infect the other during penetration or rubbing. The best advice, therefore, is to clean them before sharing.

SELF-IMAGE AND SEXUAL GROWTH

A great deal has been written on the practicalities of "safer sex." A lot of it, unfortunately, doesn't get to the heart of the matter for many people who have recently been diagnosed and are feeling very threatened by the potential changes in their sexual habits.

In the ASHA survey, for example, many respondents noted ways in which herpes affected their sense of sexual spontaneity or freedom. Some felt more hesitant to approach new partners, while a few withdrew from sexual activity for months or even years. Two out of three said they experienced a decrease in sexual pleasure around the time of diagnosis. And almost as many reported that herpes lessened sexual drive during outbreaks.

As with other aspects of genital herpes, for many individuals the impact on sexuality lessens markedly over time. In the short term, however, one may experience a sense of loss in having to feel more constrained in one's sex life. Frequently, a period of adjustment—even a period of mourning—may be needed.

At the same time, it can be very damaging to conclude that you're no longer a sexual person or no longer allowed to express sexual desire. STDs such as herpes sometimes have the seeming power to overwhelm us and become what psychologists call "defining traits." Thus, self-image can undergo a dramatic change because of a virus.

If you're feeling this way, it may be important to keep sight of the fact that millions of people with herpes do have satisfying sexual relationships. When questioned about the long-term impact of herpes, counselors and sex therapists point out that a condition like genital herpes can actually have a very positive effect on relationships. There is more to sex, they note, than intercourse. Physical affection and stimulation can take many forms. Once couples have begun to deal successfully with the emotional issue of herpes, they are often forced to explore and grow sexually. They would rather have grown without the impetus of herpes, but they have grown nonetheless.

Herpes can press couples to communicate about what is sexually pleasing. And that's no small accomplishment, because people in all sorts of relationships often have trouble talking about sex. Needs and desires remain unspoken out of embarrassment. But being forced to speak about them can have unforeseen benefits and result in more mature and more creative sex.

An easy way to begin communicating about sex is to tell your partner you want to talk about it. Talking about "talking about" sex can lead a couple to share their fears and feelings. They may then be comfortable enough to begin an ongoing process of sexual communication.

Sexual behavior is learned, not innate. People—men especially—often have learned that sexual activity must always include the genitals and penetration. These activities can be very pleasurable, but focusing exclusively on them shuts off equally enjoyable alternatives.

Sex counselors and therapists often start couples off with very general body-pleasing exercises rather than concentrating on intercourse. Through activities like sensual massage, people can begin to see the whole body as sexual. Each begins to learn what he or she enjoys and can communicate this to the partner. Once a person becomes more sophisticated about and more comfortable with sexual desires, he or she can become more satisfied in love-making.

Says one therapist: "I've had clients who have had to deal with severe herpes outbreaks over time. But it's not really an issue. A satisfying sexuality really has more to do with being comfortable with sexuality in general, being able to talk about it with your partner, and being willing to try new things with your partner. Healthy sexuality has more to do with the couple's *attitude* about sex than it has to do with an issue such as herpes."

If all the talk about condoms and spermicide puts you off, or if you've been diagnosed recently and are just not ready to become sexually active, remember two things: First, it may take a while before you feel yourself again, but you're still a whole and healthy individual who can have satisfying sexual relationships. Second, you may discover new aspects of your sexuality because of herpes.

THINKING THROUGH THE ISSUES

Faced with all this information, many people understandably

types? And will they have more frequent recurrences as a result? Calculating the odds of this is extremely complex. Here again the person with pre-existing HSV-1 infection has some protection against HSV-2. Likewise, the person with HSV-2 has protection—probably even better protection—against type 1. So the body's natural defenses are at least partially engaged. In addition, one might weigh the "sites of preference" argument—that is, even if one becomes infected with genital HSV-1, recurrences are less frequent than they are with genital HSV-2. Recurrences of oral HSV-2 are even rarer.

All the same, exposure to a sufficiently large dose of virus could result in transmission. Therefore, it's *safest* to avoid contact with lesions and to refrain from sex during outbreaks.

Another matter worth mentioning is drug therapy. If your herpes flare-ups are frequent and are posing problems in an important relationship, you might consider suppressive therapy with an antiviral drug. As noted here and in Chapter Eight, a daily dose of an antiviral drug can completely halt outbreaks in many people. The use of suppressive medication cannot guarantee you'll be completely free of subclinical shedding and should not be considered a sole form of prevention, but it can affect the pattern of recurrent outbreaks and unrecognized reactivation as well. It's something you may want to discuss with your health-care provider.

Some couples in long-term relationships find that they are less concerned about the possibility of transmission as time goes on. Some couples who have transmitted herpes after many years even report a feeling of relief, as the worry about transmitting herpes proved more troublesome than genital herpes itself. Again, how couples respond to herpes in a long-term relationship depends upon many individual factors.

In the end, genital herpes doesn't have to stand in the way of having a healthy and satisfying sex life. Taking precautions to protect your partner—and to protect yourself from other STDs—is something that more and more people are learning to negotiate. There are as many different approaches as there are different people. Just keep in mind that there is more to safer sex than latex or spermicides. Trust and communication lie at the center of any healthy relationship.

important to review the package insert or other written instructions about how to use them correctly. The basics are as follows:

• Condoms should be stored in a cool, dry place out of direct sunlight—no wallets or glove compartments.

• Put the condom on before any genital contact occurs. If the condom has a reservoir tip, squeeze the tip closed and unroll the condom onto the erect penis. Air bubbles may lead to breakage.

• If the condom does not have a reservoir tip, hold the end of the condom between the thumb and the forefinger and unroll the condom onto the erect penis. This should leave extra room at the tip of the condom (to hold the semen after ejaculation).

• Unroll the condom to cover the entire erect penis. The unrolled ring should be on the outside. If the condom is on inside out, do not flip it over. Use another one.

• *If the condom is latex*, only water-based lubricants should be used (K-Y® Brand Jelly, Replens®, or Astroglide®, for example). Oil-based lubricants can damage latex, so do not use Vaseline® petroleum jelly, baby oil, vegetable oil, or most hand and skin lotions.

• *If the condom is plastic*, the oil-based lubricants mentioned above are perfectly safe.

- Following ejaculation, while the penis is still erect,
  hold the base of the condom and withdraw, taking care
  not to let the condom slip off. A condom should never
  be used twice.

Condoms can be used for various sexual activities. They are
tested under conditions that simulate vaginal intercourse, but
experts consider them effective for oral sex and anal sex as well.
Condoms can be used with or without lubricant. Many brands
are coated with lubricant at the factory, though unlubricated
brands are also available. Because many people object to the smell
and taste of latex, some manufacturers also market flavored condoms specifically for use in oral sex.

For those who discover an allergic reaction to latex, today's
plastic condoms offer an excellent alternative.

In fact, because of the emphasis on safer sex beginning in the
late 1980s, condom manufacturers actually have been quite busy
developing new models. In addition to the plastic condom
recently developed, there are a number of condoms designed to
be used by women. One type of female condom (Reality®)
resembles a pouch with a flexible loop on either end. The smaller
of the two loops is inserted in the vagina, covering the cervix, and
the larger loop lies outside, covering the vulva. Because it covers
more area, this model might actually offer greater protection
against STDs than the standard male condom. In any case, it
gives women an option they can initiate. Some women whose
partners cannot or will not use latex condoms are able to use the
female condom.

As we noted, male condoms can be used for oral sex, but

a couple, depending on the individuals and their circumstances. The following scenarios illustrate two possibilities.

"Looking for Love"

Diane is in her mid-20s. She got herpes from someone she dated when she was just out of college. The relationship ended some time ago. She's dated a couple of people since then, but hasn't had sex with any of them. Now she's interested in Roger, and she's told him about having herpes. He still wants to get involved, but he doesn't know quite what to do about protection.

Diane suggests they shouldn't have sex when she's having an outbreak, which is three or four times a year. Also, she has lived with her herpes long enough that she knows exactly when an outbreak is coming on, so she's never caught by surprise. But she wonders about unrecognized herpes reactivation.

She also wonders about Roger's past history. He's had several partners before Diane, and he's never been tested for any sexually transmitted infection.

After considering the risks for both of them, they decide they will become sexually intimate, but they choose to use condoms every time they're together and to refrain from sex when Diane has symptoms.

THE CHARACTERS HERE could be younger or middle-aged, straight, gay, or bisexual. With HIV around, however, there is good reason to know your partner's sexual history, and good reason to use condoms.

Of course, there are also are situations in which people don't make choices as a couple and may not have the benefit of knowing a partner's past history. In the proverbial "one-night stand," a person is well-advised to use condoms or practice some form of safer sex. The choice to "just take the risk" and ignore the need for protection is often one that people come to regret.

THE STEADY RELATIONSHIP

Back to Diane and Roger. They're still together a year later, and have decided to move in together. They both want the relationship to last, and they figure it probably will. Roger has begun to question why they're using condoms. He's seen that Diane has very little problem with herpes, and he wonders whether it's worth the trouble of taking precautions between outbreaks. So they talk about it. Diane says she's not worried about getting an STD from Roger, and they trust each other. Still, they feel it would be best if they both get checked out for some of the other sexually transmitted diseases that can hang around for years but cause no symptoms.

In the end, they both get a "clean bill of health," and they decide together that they'll stop using condoms in between outbreaks, but put off sex when symptoms are present. They know there is some risk with herpes, but they're in love, and they're willing to take it.

THERE ARE MANY possible variations here, of course. Roger may have been determined to avoid getting herpes, or Diane may have been determined to avoid transmitting it, and therefore they may have preferred to stick with condoms. Or either partner may

Among those who find herpes troubling, some look for alternatives in managing the infection, often because of the expense or the inconvenience of prescription medications, or because, like Nate, they have philosophical objections to them. Instead, they look for other ways to take control.

Nate's solution, dietary vitamin supplements, is one of the myriad approaches proposed or questioned by people writing and calling the Herpes Resource Center. There are advocates for acupuncture, Chinese medicine, chiropractic, dietary changes, herbal remedies, homeopathy, hypnosis, naturopathy, psychotherapy, group therapy, 12-step groups, visualization, and more.

The list is long, and it grows each year. The movement toward alternative medicine, in fact, is a national trend of considerable scope. Based on a 1991 survey, one out of every three Americans has experimented with an alternative treatment of some kind, and we collectively spend $27 billion a year in the process. Partly as a result, the National Institutes of Health has now set up a special branch to study alternative medicine.

Unfortunately, until some of these studies are completed, it's difficult to evaluate alternative therapies for herpes. The fact is that most are not scientifically tested and retested the way that prescription drugs are scrutinized. In the vast majority of cases, there are no "double-blind" studies, so one can never be sure that the results would have appeared the same to an unconvinced observer. These therapies also lack an approval process that hinges on the performance of a given treatment in a large cross-section of people. What we're left with in most cases are the personal accounts of a few individuals who have tried something, found it successful for them, and either want to share what they've learned or find out whether the approach is medically safe.

Because ASHA is asked about many of these treatments, we wish we were in a better position to broker solid information. Sadly, we don't have much hard evidence about many of the alternative therapies suggested. We can, however, share what we know about the approaches most commonly used by people with recurrent genital herpes.

WHAT TRIGGERS HERPES?

It's not exactly an "alternative therapy," perhaps, but probably the most common approach to managing recurrent herpes is to try to identify and avoid the things most likely to bring on an outbreak.

What are the so-called triggers that cause HSV to break out of its latent phase and become active again? Over the years, people with herpes have put forth many candidates. These include sickness, psychological stress, fatigue, menstruation, and poor nutrition. Sun exposure—even the mildest sunburn—can be a trigger for HSV, as can irritation or friction at the site of infection. For some, vigorous sex can cause this kind of irritation.

The 1991 ASHA survey found a similar ranking of likely trigger factors. In all, over 70% of respondents agreed that "stressful events contribute to herpes symptoms." Asked to check off specific factors that seem to bring on herpes outbreaks, 49% cited crisis or strain in a relationship and 30% chose problems at work. But many of the factors centered on physical stresses, such as lack of sleep (38%), sexual activity (37%), and illness (33%). Some 19% blamed flare-ups on poor nutrition, and 11% targeted lack of exercise. Among women, 52% cited menstruation as a probable trigger.

Few of these possible triggers have been closely studied by researchers, but some work has been done. Scientists have noted several types of outbreak stimulants in lab animals, among them: skin irritation at the site of infection, surgical trauma to the nerve or ganglion where the latent virus resides, and radiation.

Recently, very detailed studies have looked at the role of intense ultraviolet light on facial cold sores caused by HSV-1. In these studies, 70% of the subjects exposed to about two hours of midday sun developed herpes symptoms within a week. But subjects who used sunscreen were protected. The message for people who get cold sores is clear, particularly if they're sensitive to the sun. On the basis of a few small research studies, it seems that ultraviolet light may well have a similar effect in triggering genital herpes in those who have prolonged and direct exposures of the buttocks or genital area.

Menstruation remains prominent as a trigger factor in anecdotal accounts, but researchers have not found evidence of this in controlled studies.

CAN YOU AVOID PHYSICAL TRIGGERS?

From a strictly scientific point of view, outbreaks cannot be predicted with accuracy. No one will be able to identify the certain cause of every flare-up, and some people won't have a clue about any of them. At the same time, however, it appears that most people with herpes do begin to associate certain events or behaviors with reactivation.

Once identified, triggers can *sometimes* be avoided. If sunburn gives you a bad case of cold sores, there is always sunscreen, lip balm, and a hat. If outbreaks are brought on by a lack of sleep, maybe it's time to get serious about a quality eight hours every night. If drinking too much coffee or alcohol puts you on the ragged edge of a recurrence, there is the choice between moderation and paying the consequences.

The solutions aren't always simple, of course, and we want to emphasize that none of these approaches is likely to give you total control over HSV. Many triggers are not known or can't be foreseen. Others you may have good reason to suspect but can't do much about. The last thing you want to do is blame yourself for recurrences or try endless experimental strategies to avoid them. For some, this becomes another form of obsession.

If, on the other hand, you gain clear insight into your pattern of outbreaks, you may find practical ways of sometimes averting them. Over time your knowledge of your own triggers and your sensitivity to prodromal symptoms will likely increase. This information, in turn, is something you can use in defining your own coping strategies, with or without the use of antiviral drugs.

PSYCHOLOGICAL STRESS

Over two-thirds of the respondents in ASHA's 1991 survey indicated that "stressful events contribute to herpes symptoms." Behavorial research on the subject, however, is inconclusive.

So what's to be done about it? As we suggest in the preceding section on physical stresses, there is little point for most of us in trying to create "stress-free" lives. In fact, even if we did, there is no proof that we'd be free from HSV reactivations.

On the other hand, there are several well-known techniques for managing stress, and some people with herpes report that they are helpful. Biofeedback, meditation, hypnosis, visualization, regular exercise, psychotherapy—all these and more have been employed successfully by some individuals. There are no cumulative statistics on success rates for most of these, though biofeedback and relaxation training have perhaps the most credible research support across a range of stress-related disorders. There is also one published study on visualization which claims that people using this technique for herpes experienced gains similar to those of people in support groups.

EMOTIONAL SUPPORT

One persuasive behavioral study suggests that people with genital herpes can best manage anxiety over recurrences if they get "herpes-specific social support." In other words, while some amount of stress is inevitable, people can devise more effective ways of managing it. And some researchers believe that stress is less likely to trigger a herpes outbreak if you can talk to someone about herpes and rely on his or her emotional support when you need it. Usually, the researchers found, this support came from a spouse or lover, but it could also come from a close friend or family member. People with these kinds of relationships were not stress-free, but they had fewer outbreaks.

We already have spoken at length in this book about the benefits of putting herpes "on the table" in intimate relationships. If you don't have this kind of relationship at the moment, or if you have become socially isolated because of herpes, involvement in a support group may help you to put herpes in perspective and break the pattern of withdrawal from others.

Around 1980, in the well-publicized heyday of the genital herpes epidemic, ASHA's Herpes Resource Center fostered the creation of local support groups (HELP Groups) in cities around the United States. Many of these groups have flourished for more than a decade under local volunteer leadership, helping individuals make emotional adjustments in the wake of a herpes diagnosis and get their lives back on track.

"It's a diverse mix of people that participates," writes Paul in the newsletter of one group. "In the beginning, we start out as strangers. And the fascinating thing about the group is the degree of honesty with which we communicate. This honesty builds trust. Friendships form quickly. The thing that has slowed us down for so long expedites the development of our relationships."

"My 18 months of isolation were finally at an end," says a former member of another local HELP Group. "These people were the first I'd known who shared the illness and could speak freely with me about it. There was a great deal of humor to the sessions as well. This was part of the healing. I do not consider it a coincidence that the frequency and intensity of my outbreaks had dropped considerably by the time I left the group."

We certainly do not want to imply by these testimonials that going to a support group is guaranteed to keep herpes in check— nor is it necessary for everyone. Depending on your own personality and the nature of the group, you may get only modest gains from it. But for thousands of people each year, the local groups

not alone. The one area of general agreement seems to be this: If your diet is inadequate in some way, this can definitely have a negative effect on your health and your resistance to infections. Seeking help from a nutritionist may be a good idea. He or she probably will not be able to control herpes specifically with dietary changes, but the benefits to your health as a whole may carry over to herpes.

NONCONVENTIONAL REMEDIES

Beyond the vitamins, minerals, and amino acids of a balanced diet, there remains a good deal of interest in specific remedies. Goldenseal, for example, is an herb that is thought to have antiviral properties, and some people use it for herpes, either in capsules or strong teas. Garlic, an ancient folk remedy for colds, has been shown to inhibit a number of viruses and bacteria in the laboratory, herpes among them. Some people, therefore, take garlic in capsules, and they report good results. Practitioners of homeopathic medicine, naturopathic medicine, and Chinese herbal medicine also have treatments for people with herpes. We wish we could say more about these approaches, but they simply haven't been rigorously tested in large numbers of people.

There also can be health risks associated with herpes remedies. Some people, for example, have used dye-light therapy for herpes, a practice that can cause cancerous changes in healthy cells. And many topical creams or oils—even over-the-counter products such as cortisone creams—will actually slow the healing of herpes lesions.

It's also worth considering that some alternative therapies, even megadoses of vitamins, are quite costly. If you have frequent outbreaks, antiviral therapy may give you significantly more benefit for your drugstore dollar than nutritional supplements or herbal remedies.

Learning more about the pros and cons of alternative therapies is not easy, but the coming years should bring us more information about the safety and effectiveness of various approaches.

THE "HEALTHY LIFESTYLE"

Each of us might have a different definition of the healthy lifestyle, but there seems to be broad agreement that, regardless of herpes, certain behaviors help keep us operating at peak performance. These include: eating a balanced diet, getting the proper amount of sleep and exercise, avoiding excesses of caffeine and alcohol, staying away from tobacco, and being careful to manage chronic stress. Medical science has had a lot to say about the benefits of these "lifestyle choices" as they apply to cancer, heart disease, and various other important health problems.

Many sing the praises of the healthy lifestyle when it comes to herpes, as well. "Herpes has really forced me to look at my life and set priorities," says one woman. "Now I watch what I eat, get plenty of sleep, and have become an avid jogger. I feel so much better, and my outbreaks seem to be less and less a problem."

As in the case of alternative medicines, the comments generally are not based on rigorous science. But the basic health lessons of childhood—beginning with "eat your vegetables"— seem to hold merit for lots of people.

In a way, you might regard herpes as you would the common

cold. You know that your body is constantly challenged by various germs. But even when there is a cold "going around" your family or your office, your immune system often protects you. Then, if you lose sleep or just get generally "run down," suddenly you've lost the battle and you've got that cold. The object of the healthy lifestyle is precisely this: Don't run that body down.

14

HERPES AND PREGNANCY

"After having several outbreaks a year, I got pregnant with my first child," writes Marilu. "And deep down I was really worried—childbirth was the one thing about herpes that always seemed scary to me. Even so, despite tremendous stress during pregnancy (change of jobs, and moving) I had only one outbreak. I delivered vaginally after a long and painful labor. My baby and I were treated with kind and loving care, and after a two-day stay, we went home. My next outbreak occurred a month later."

Even people who have learned to manage genital herpes with ease sometimes have concerns about pregnancy and their ability to give birth to a healthy child. On one hand, these worries are reasonable, because HSV infection in a newborn can be a devastating illness. On the other hand, this kind of herpes infection is quite rare. Out of approximately 4 million live births every year in the United States, an estimated 3,000-4,000 babies contract neonatal herpes. In many cases, these babies are born to women who contract herpes late in pregnancy, rather than to women who have long-standing infections. What's more, women who have genital herpes and recognize it can take precautions to lower the already small risk that their infants might become infected.

HOW HSV CAN SPREAD TO NEWBORNS

Transmission of genital HSV to newborns follows the same basic principles that govern transmission between adults. It's just that the contact between infant and mother's genitals is most likely to occur during labor and delivery. If HSV reactivates in a pregnant woman during labor, it's likely that she will be shedding virus somewhere in the birth canal. Visible herpes lesions pose the greatest threat to the infant. Asymptomatic shedding also poses some risk, mainly if it occurs as part of a first episode.

While the vast majority of transmission from mother to infant takes place at birth, there are two other possibilities. First, researchers believe that in very rare cases a fetus may become infected during pregnancy if the mother has a severe primary episode. The theory here is that there is a large amount of HSV present in the mother's system, and some of it may cross the placenta or find its way into the amniotic fluid through tiny self-healing leaks in the amniotic sac. Secondly, some infants become infected after birth if an adult with active herpes lesions transmits HSV through direct contact. The classic example of this is the relative who has an active cold sore and kisses a baby.

ASSESSING THE RISK

Research on neonatal herpes conducted during the late 1980s has shed a great deal of light on the question of which deliveries carry the highest risk. It turns out that more than half of the babies infected with herpes at delivery are born to mothers who are having primary or first episodes of genital herpes in the last few weeks of pregnancy. In this situation, the risk of transmission

HERPES AND PREGNANCY

can be as high as 30% to 40%. Some of these women actually had herpes lesions but were not adequately examined before giving birth. Others may have been shedding virus asymptomatically as a result of a first episode. If this seems hard to believe, remember that most people with genital HSV-2 don't know they carry the virus. People are capable of transmitting herpes through sex without knowing it; likewise they are capable of infecting an infant.

In rare cases, babies also can become infected when exposed to asymptomatic viral shedding in the birth canal of mothers who have recurrent genital herpes. In this situation, the risk of transmission to a newborn is quite small—probably much less than 1%. When a mother with recurrent herpes has an outbreak at the time of delivery, the risk is much less than with a first episode, but it's considered high enough that medical experts recommend delivery by cesarean section (C-section). Prematurity may increase the risk to the newborn.

Why are the differences between each class of herpes infection so dramatic? A primary or first episode raises the level of risk for four reasons: Neither mother nor infant will have antibodies to HSV, because it's a first-time exposure. More virus is present in a first episode than in a recurrent outbreak. The cervix is more often involved, which means the baby has a higher probability of coming into contact with virus in the birth canal. And the virus remains active for a longer period.

Babies born to women with recurrent genital herpes, on the other hand, have a major advantage. Nature offers significant protection to these infants by giving them HSV antibodies while they're still in the womb. These antibodies come directly from

mend them for similar reasons. The fear of malpractice suits also contributes to the high rate of C-sections among women with genital herpes.

The problem is that C-sections themselves carry a substantial risk and a high cost. A C-section is major surgery that entails the health risks of anesthesia, costs several thousand dollars more than a vaginal delivery, and involves a longer and more complicated period of recovery.

In planning your baby's delivery, it's also important to learn about the policies of the hospital or birthing center you plan to use. Certain hospitals have very strict procedures for isolating patients whose pregnancy is complicated by an infectious disease such as herpes. Some women have complained of offensive and backward procedures, including quarantining mothers and babies—even when neither mother nor baby has symptoms of active infection. If you have a C-section that is officially justified on the basis of "genital herpes," you may find that the hospital will apply special rules to you and your baby. This might affect plans you have for rooming-in, for example. Not all institutions will have such rules, but it's a good idea to know in advance if yours does. What you learn may also raise the question of choosing a different hospital, since these sorts of isolation policies are no longer recommended by experts in the field.

Many women wonder about the advisability of taking an antiviral drug during pregnancy to suppress outbreaks in the third trimester. No drug against herpes has been approved for this purpose by the U.S. Food and Drug Administration. Nonetheless, some doctors might use acyclovir to treat women who have a primary episode during pregnancy. In one small study, women with first episodes during pregnancy took daily acyclovir during the third trimester and were able to suppress reactivation effectively. None of the women taking daily antiviral medication was delivered by C-section, versus 36% of the place-bo group.

It should be noted that acyclovir markedly reduces asympto-matic shedding as well as outbreaks in women who aren't preg-nant. However, women in late pregnancy are immunosuppressed, and their bodies may not respond to acyclovir the same way. One theoretical possibility is that in pregnant women with recurrent genital herpes, acyclovir would simply modify symptoms, so that the woman wouldn't realize that she was having an outbreak. More studies on this issue are likely.

In addition to the cases in which acyclovir has been pre-scribed during pregnancy, some women have used it inadvertently before they realized they were expecting. So far, a voluntary reg-istry that tracks both kinds of patients—more than 1000 at this writing—has seen no indication that the drug is harmful to mother or child. Still, there is not enough evidence to pronounce the drug categorically safe in pregnancy.

One other issue worth mentioning centers on labor itself. This is the use of fetal scalp monitors. In the largest study to date on herpes and pregnancy, researchers at the University of Washington found that use of this type of monitor appeared to increase the risk of infection. The reason, probably, is that these instruments cause a tiny puncture in the fetus's scalp, offering a possible opening for virus to enter. The study results weren't con-clusive, but experts believe that for women with a history of geni-tal herpes, fetal scalp monitors should be used only when

skin at all. Typically, however, herpes symptoms develop within several days to two weeks. These can include the classic herpes lesions seen in adults, red swollen eyes (conjunctivitis), general irritability, lack of interest in food, jaundice, pneumonia, and convulsions.

Because the initial symptoms of herpes infection overlap with those of more common childhood illnesses, diagnosis can be quite difficult. Viral culture is often used as a diagnostic test. For quicker and more accurate diagnosis, there is the prospect that a DNA test called "polymerase chain reaction" (PCR) will be perfected for HSV and widely used in the near future.

The severity of herpes in newborns varies greatly. If infection is confined to the skin, eyes, and mouth, the infant's prognosis is usually good. But sometimes in newborns the virus can infect the blood and spread widely. In another frequent complication, herpes can attack the brain (encephalitis), causing irreversible damage.

With any form of neonatal infection, early diagnosis and treatment are critical. Acyclovir is effective in many cases. Some doctors will start an infant on acyclovir even before a herpes diagnosis is confirmed, provided there is strong suspicion that HSV is the cause of the child's illness. But this strategy is a controversial one in medical circles. Some doctors also will treat an infant if the mother had a first episode during a vaginal delivery, because the chances of transmission in this situation are so high. Researchers are testing new approaches as well. In the area of therapy, researchers are testing the idea that infants who were exposed to HSV at birth might benefit from a dose of HSV antibodies or a combination of antibodies and an antiviral drug.

PROTECTING THE BABY AT HOME

Even when a baby is born without herpes, it's important to remember that there is still a risk of infection, and herpes can be a very serious illness in the first few weeks of life. Accordingly, mothers and fathers with active herpes sores should take care to protect their babies. If you're having an outbreak (or even if you're not), some logical precautions include the following:

- Wash your hands before touching the baby.

- If a visiting friend or relative has a cold sore, warn him or her about the risks of spreading HSV to your newborn through a kiss.

- Wear a mask if you have sores on the mouth (to keep you from inadvertently touching the mouth and then the baby).

The point here is not to discourage all of the touching and cuddling that commonly go along with taking care of a newborn. These kinds of contact are very necessary. But if you're having an outbreak, safety is an important concern, and you'll want to take steps to keep the child away from direct contact with places where virus is present on the skin.

WHAT YOU CAN DO

Many of the decisions about managing herpes at delivery call for discussion with your doctor or midwife. Be sure to tell your

tions here, we run the risk of scaring the reader with what may sound like irrelevant information. If ASHA were creating a book for drivers' education, this would be like including a whole chapter on what to do in the event that all four tires go flat at one time.

All the same, we do want this book to serve as a useful information resource. We think it's important, therefore, to establish some basic facts about herpes complications, and to quash some of the misinformation currently spread.

HERPES WHITLOW

Among the forms of "autoinoculation" already mentioned, herpes of the fingers (herpes whitlow) deserves further explanation because it can occur in a number of ways. Generally, whitlow results when virus is spread to a finger that has a cut or abrasion. Once there, it can cause an outbreak with symptoms similar to those of oral-facial or genital herpes. These outbreaks may also recur.

First, of course, the virus has to get to the finger. In people who have genital herpes, this is most likely to occur through autoinoculation during a primary episode, as was explained earlier (Chapter Three). Many cases of whitlow, however, have been traced to adults who have HSV-1 on the mouth or face and who have the habit of biting their fingernails. Active HSV-1 can deposit virus in saliva, and the biting can create an opening in the skin that allows HSV a portal of entry.

In the past, herpes whitlow also has afflicted significant numbers of dentists, surgeons, and other health-care professionals whose hands are frequently in contact with patients' saliva. In

recent years, however, the use of latex hand gloves and other precautions appears to have reduced the incidence of whitlow in
health-care workers, and today, most whitlow is caused by HSV-2
in sexually active adults.

For this reason, people with active herpes lesions are advised
to avoid touching them. If you do make contact, it's best to wash
the hands right away. Soap and water will kill the virus and avert
risk of whitlow. And if you have oral-facial herpes, remember:
Biting the nails may be risky.

OCULAR HERPES

Ocular herpes, meaning an infection of the eye, is almost
always caused by HSV-1, although the source of infection in
infants is usually HSV-2. In rare cases, ocular herpes is linked to
autoinoculation, but typically eye infection occurs when latent
HSV-1 reactivates and simply travels to the eye instead of the
mouth or lips. Ocular infections also can be the site of a primary
type 1 infection.

Symptoms sometimes begin with blisters or cold sores on the
eyelid and the itchy, watery sort of "pink eye" associated with
conjunctivitis. Later symptoms typically include pain and sensitivity to light. If left untreated, ocular herpes can lead to increasingly painful lesions on the cornea. Some cases resolve by themselves and don't recur, though the majority of patients will have a
second episode at some point. Recurrent ocular infections must
be treated with antiviral medication; otherwise, they can ultimately damage the structure of the eye, leading to impaired vision. A
variety of treatments are available, including topical trifluridine,

with normal immune function but in up to 5% of people with AIDS. For this reason, medications such as intravenous foscarnet or the topicals cidofovir and trifluridine, which have a different way of attacking HSV, are sometimes used instead.

It's also possible—though uncommon—for people with compromised immune systems to experience what the medical literature calls "disseminated infection." This means the virus may move in unanticipated directions, reaching internal organs such as the lungs or the liver and stomach. Newborns who become infected with herpes are sometimes afflicted by this condition.

To return to the question that opened this chapter, do people with herpes have to worry about donating blood? The answer is no, unless they are in the midst of a *true primary* episode. The reason is that a small amount of virus may get into the blood at this time. Therefore, we advise that people with true primary outbreaks refrain from donating blood for two reasons: First of all, you're unwell just now, and it doesn't make any sense to weaken yourself further by losing blood. In fact, donating blood is not recommended for persons with flu or any other "acute illness." Second, there is the remote possibility of virus being present in the blood.

What about the guidelines for those with *recurrent* genital herpes? Experts actually do not recommend donating blood *during outbreaks*, because it's a further strain on the body. Otherwise, people with recurrent genital herpes *do not* have to worry about spreading the virus when they donate blood. There is no documented case of HSV ever having been spread from a blood transfusion, and blood banks do not routinely screen for HSV.

THE BOTTOM LINE

For people who have genital herpes, there is wisdom in taking precautions to avoid the problem of autoinoculation. Anyone having a first episode would be well-advised to avoid touching lesions if possible, and to wash the hands immediately if the fingers do rub against herpes sores. This simple step can avert many cases of whitlow in adults, which is largely preventable, and a small number of ocular herpes cases, as well.

As for the rest, remember that complications such as disseminated HSV infection are most likely to appear in people with a compromised immune system. If you are undergoing cancer treatment that will suppress your immune function, for example, you would be well-advised to tell your doctor about a history of herpes so that prophylactic antiviral therapy can be considered. The same advice goes for people who are newly diagnosed with HIV: For those with many or severe outbreaks, suppressive therapy is often used.

in herpes diagnostics is the virus culture test. With this method, the doctor takes a swab and uses it to pick up cells from an active herpes lesion. The swab, which has now picked up a small quantity of virus, is carefully packed into a special solution and sent to the laboratory. At the lab, the virus from the swab is allowed to grow for several days in a collection of cells from healthy human skin tissue or other sources. If HSV is indeed present on the swab, it will cause certain changes in the cell culture that can be spotted easily under a microscope. A confirmatory test should be used as well, to verify that the cell changes are truly due to herpes. In essence, the virus culture test transplants the virus into another setting and allows it to grow until its effects on cells are visible.

The major advantage of the virus culture test is its accuracy. The culture has *specificity*, meaning it will not be positive for herpes if another organism is causing the lesions.

This is not to say that the culture test always works or has no drawbacks. The samples for virus culture must be taken when virus can be found on the surface of the skin or of mucous membranes such as the vagina. The best samples, then, are taken from lesions that contain large amounts of virus—those that have not yet had a chance to crust or scab. If the lesions are in the process of healing, the culture test often yields a "false negative" result; that is, the swab won't pick up enough virus and the test will fail to find HSV, even though the virus really is the culprit. The culture test is most likely (80% to 90%) to be positive during first episodes, when large amounts of virus are present. It is less likely to be positive during recurrences, with a detection rate of only 30% to 60%.

Another potential disadvantage to this test is that it often takes many hours before cellular changes occur in the culture medium, so the results are anything but rapid. Most lab reports will take from two to seven days.

Waiting for the results may require patience, but in many cases this is an effort worth making; the virus culture test is still the most reliable tool around for an initial herpes diagnosis. The test costs anywhere from $40 to $100 (depending on the lab chosen), not including the cost of an office visit. If the results are negative and your health-care provider has good reason to suspect HSV anyway, he or she will probably ask you to come back to the office promptly the next time you have an outbreak, so that a better sample can be obtained.

OTHER COMMON DIAGNOSTIC TOOLS

Among the alternatives to cell culture, the most impressive challenger at the moment is a test that identifies HSV "antigens," virus particles that provoke the immune system to respond. This procedure begins the same way a virus culture does: The doctor uses a swab to get virus from an active lesion. The lab then combines this sample with HSV antibodies and a "detector system." Detector systems can be enzymes which cause color changes or fluorescence if HSV antigens are present in the specimen.

Because antigen test kits don't require HSV to replicate and grow, the test is faster than a culture, taking only a few hours (though results will seldom be reported back from the lab this quickly). The test also rates well in the area of specificity. It rarely confuses HSV with something else. In terms of cost, it's generally in the same range as the cell culture, though prices fluc-

negative in a viral culture?

One diagnostic tool that skirts the problem of sampling active lesions is the blood test, properly called a "serologic assay" by medical experts. Serologic tests detect antibodies to HSV that your body continually supplies to your blood stream. Beginning just a few weeks after infection with HSV, these antibodies can be searched out at any time, regardless of whether HSV is in its active or latent phase. Their presence certifies infection.

So far, so good. The downfall of most serologies, however, is distinguishing HSV-1 from HSV-2. Because 50% to 80% of the adult population has HSV-1 already, these tests typically aren't very useful in identifying genital herpes. That is, the test result will indicate the presence of herpes antibody, but it's often hard to know whether or not this antibody reflects long-standing HSV-1 infection in the facial area. In many cases, it probably does.

Many serologies claim to be "type-specific," and lab reports will show a reading separately for type 1 and type 2. Unfortunately, though, most serologic tests will "cross-react" with antibodies for either viral type (or sometimes with other herpesviruses). What shows up as type 2 may really be type 1, and vice versa. So the results are often worthless.

Does this mean it's best to write off serologies altogether? No. Bona fide tests that are truly type-specific do exist. With these, patients can know for certain what researchers call their "serostatus"—that is, do they have HSV-1, HSV-2, neither, or both? And patients can know this whether they have symptomatic outbreaks or not.

Already these tests have been used to prove the extent of herpes infection among adults, to shed light on the existence of viral shedding when no lesions are present, and to show that HSV-1 provides some form of natural defense against HSV-2. In studies ranging from HSV and pregnancy outcome to experimental vaccines, the type-specific serology is an increasingly indispensable tool for understanding the intricacies of the virus.

The "gold standard" for HSV serologies is the Western blot, developed by the Virology Laboratory at the University of Washington in Seattle. In addition, accurate type-specific HSV serologies should become commercially available through doctor's offices and clinics soon. The National Herpes Hotline provides updates (see page 195). However, a serology is not a first-line diagnostic tool such as a cell culture or antigen test. For one thing, it doesn't reveal the site of infection: If you have HSV-1, for example, is it genital or facial?

Though the test has its limitations, the new generation of type-specific serologies may prove invaluable to people with herpes in several ways. Take, for example, the problem of averting herpes in the newborn. The greatest danger of neonatal herpes occurs when the mother is experiencing a first episode of herpes late in pregnancy. So the problem becomes one of identifying the women at highest risk. Remember Phil and Carla from Chapter Fourteen? Carla is pregnant. A type-specific serology for her and her husband Phil might reveal that she has neither HSV-1 nor HSV-2, but that Phil has HSV-2. She is at high risk, therefore, of contracting herpes and then transmitting it to her baby. In this case, it would be wise for the couple to use condoms throughout pregnancy, or take other precautions to keep Phil from infecting Carla at this critical time.

VACCINE RESEARCH

The most dramatic developments at the moment are taking place in the arena of vaccine research. Scientists are experimenting with several different approaches to "immunize" a person against herpes simplex.

A herpes vaccine could work in much the same way that traditional immunizations do. These protect a person against future infection by exposing the body to a small amount of the target germ, so that the immune system has a chance to set up its defenses against the invader. The body then retains a long-term ability to defeat this particular germ. As a result, the person who gets vaccinated remains healthy.

With HSV specifically, a vaccine would first and foremost protect a person who is not yet infected. Once immunized, a person might be exposed to HSV repeatedly and never become sick, because the immune system would be fully armed and prepared to hold herpes in check. Ideally, the vaccine would prevent a person from becoming infected with HSV-2. Of less benefit, at least one vaccine now in development would not prevent an uninfected person from acquiring HSV-2, but would prevent or lower the number of symptomatic outbreaks the virus causes.

In addition, at least some of the vaccines now being tested for HSV might also help a person who is already infected. How? The vaccine might actually amplify the immune response to HSV to such a point that a person who already has genital herpes will get fewer or milder outbreaks. And there is, of course, the emotional boost of knowing that one's partner can be protected if he or she, too, is immunized. Vaccines, then, address the single most important concern of people with herpes: infecting a partner.

Fundamentally, there are two distinct approaches to an HSV vaccine. The first is the "live virus" approach, in which scientists use the whole virus but alter its genetic make-up so that it cannot cause permanent infection. This class of vaccines generally has the advantage of triggering the most dramatic immune response. But there is a disadvantage, too: A live-virus immunization could carry a *chance* of causing disease and becoming latent. It's usually a small chance, but this risk has to be carefully considered with herpesviruses.

The second approach uses an "inactivated" virus vaccine. For this, researchers employ either a "killed virus" or isolated fragments of virus that stimulate the body's natural defenses. These vaccines do not cause disease, but they are usually less powerful in stirring up an immune response.

Researchers in dozens of laboratories around the world are pursuing numerous variations on these two basic themes. Some are using HSV-1 as the basis of the vaccine, and some HSV-2. Some are even using a distinct "third-party" virus as the vehicle, but combining it with elements of HSV.

The formulation that has been most aggressively explored is based on the inactivated virus approach described above. For this, researchers have identified specific fragments called "glycoproteins" on the surface of the herpes simplex virus. These glycoproteins play a key role in stimulating the immune response to HSV. When they're mixed in a formula with other ingredients that tend to bolster the immune defense generally, they create high levels of antibody to HSV and also activate the cellular immune response.

Unfortunately, the first major clinical trials for the glycoprotein vaccine failed to prevent transmission in discordant couples.

in the realm of biomedical research. If you have herpes, and you're anxious to hear about important scientific advances, there are any number of medical journals and texts that report on new developments. Many of these are summarized for lay audiences in *the helper*, a quarterly journal of the American Social Health Association. (See the Resource List on page 195 for details.)

18

HERPES, HIV, AND
THE OTHER STDS

Other sexually transmitted infections can be more important than herpes when discussing issues of sexual health with a partner. So it's useful to inform yourself about the broader epidemic of STDs and the steps that people can take to prevent these infections.

Each year, according to the Centers for Disease Control and Prevention (CDC), there are *12 million new sexually transmitted infections*. Some of these are caused by bacteria and are easily cured, while some, like genital herpes, are lifelong viral infections. The most common STDs include the following:

CHLAMYDIA. A bacterium, *Chlamydia trachomatis* infects an estimated 4 million Americans each year. Antibiotics will rid the body of chlamydia in a matter of days, but often the people who carry this infection fail to get prompt treatment because they have no idea they're infected. The reason is that chlamydia causes no signs or symptoms of illness in up to 75% of women and 50% of men. When there are symptoms, these often include painful urination in men, or a vaginal discharge in women.

but there is a vaccine that can prevent infection. People who contract hepatitis B may have liver damage and increased risk for liver cancer. They may carry the virus for the rest of their lives. The Centers for Disease Control and Prevention recommends vaccination for all infants, adolescents, and sexually active adults.

HIV/AIDS. You may know more about HIV/AIDS already than we can possibly cover here, but it's nevertheless important to include. HIV is, after all, transmitted primarily through unprotected sexual intercourse. So the precautions required for other STDs can help to prevent the spread of HIV, too.

As with so many other viral infections, symptoms may not show up for years after the virus takes hold. And the symptoms are extremely diverse, mimicking dozens of other illnesses. HIV attacks the immune system itself, wrecking the body's natural defenses against a host of different infections. There are treatments to slow the viral assault against the immune system, but as yet none suppress it completely.

WHILE THESE are the most troublesome STDs in many ways, others are worth mentioning as well. Common parasites such as *Trichomonas vaginalis*, frequently the cause of vaginitis (inflammation of the vaginal tissue), are often transmitted sexually—to the tune of 3 million infections annually. There are a dozen other infections easily spread through intimate contact, including sex. These include scabies and lice.

If you want more information about any or all sexually transmitted infections, there are a number of resources to call on. Two major sources of help are free of charge and as convenient as the nearest telephone. The National STD Hotline and National AIDS Hotline both offer confidential information and referrals, including print materials sent free of charge to your home address. (See Resource List, page 195.) Either hotline also can tell you the location of an STD clinic run by the public health department in your community. Testing and treatment for STDs is often free or inexpensive.

AN OUNCE OF PREVENTION

When we live amidst so many epidemic STDs, what's most critical is learning how to minimize the risk of either getting or spreading these diseases. There are some differences in how particular STDs are transmitted, but a few principles of prevention apply equally to almost all of them:

- Your risk of getting an STD is zero if you don't have sex.

- If you're free of infection yourself, your risk also is zero if you have sex only with one *uninfected* partner, who in turn has sex only with you. As soon as either partner has a new sexual contact, however, all bets are off. The catch is: With so many STDs that show no symptoms, how do you know who is infected and who isn't?

- What if you don't really know your partner well and certainly don't know about his or her past? Those having sex with a partner who *might* be carrying an STD, or with several such partners, can dramatically reduce their risk of getting or spreading an STD by using condoms for each and every act of sexual intercourse—whether the penetration is oral, vaginal, or anal. Condoms used in this way are very effective prevention for chlamydia, gonorrhea, syphilis, hepatitis B, and HIV. For STDs spread through direct contact with skin lesions, such as herpes and HPV, condoms offer less thorough protection.

• Spermicides may provide additional protection against sexually transmitted infections, but should be used along with condoms—not in place of them.

IS HERPES A PRECURSOR?

Some people with herpes question whether they are at greater risk of getting other illnesses because of HSV. Some assume that a person with one virus in the herpes family will be prone to get all of them. Others have seen press coverage which implies that herpes might somehow mutate into the AIDS virus, or that herpes itself will damage the immune system.

On all of these points, the facts should be reassuring. Because all the herpesviruses are quite common, you may host herpes simplex and several other members of the family as well, such as Epstein-Barr and varicella zoster. But having HSV in no way dooms you to getting all the herpesviruses; each one is transmitted separately. Nor does having HSV mean that you have a deficient immune system.

Lastly, herpes does not turn into HIV, although it may make a person more susceptible to contracting HIV.

Several of the other STDs mentioned in this chapter are also considered risk factors for HIV. Chlamydia, gonorrhea, syphilis—the presence of any of these infections increases the risk of acquiring HIV, *if and when* there is sexual contact with an HIV-infected person. But none of them by itself leads to HIV. (By the way, it's probable that a person with HIV is more infectious if he or she has another STD as well.)

There is also what some experts call a "behavioral" linkage between HIV and other sexually transmitted infections. In other words, if you already have an STD, there is a good chance you had unprotected sex with others who have had unprotected sex. Therefore, in statistical terms, anyone with an STD is in a high-risk group for HIV. It's important to note that alcohol use also may be considered a risk factor for HIV and other STDs, since alcohol can cloud judgment and lead to unprotected sex. These generalizations may or may not apply to you personally, but they are worth considering seriously. If you have doubts about your HIV status you can learn more about testing by calling the National AIDS Hotline.

WHAT YOU CAN DO

If you have herpes, you now know that sexually transmitted infections are real and present in your life as well as in millions of other lives. Call the National STD Hotline for more information about STDs, for free written materials, or to get a referral to a health-care provider in your community. If you feel you may have been exposed to other STDs through unprotected sex, or if you have symptoms that resemble those of a common STD, talk to your health-care provider about it. There are screening tests for all the infections listed here. And as always, early treatment is the key to avoiding serious medical complications.

19

LEGAL ISSUES

"I was dating this girl, and we slept together once," says a caller to the National Herpes Hotline. "Now I've got herpes, and I'm thinking about taking legal action. I'm sure I got it from her. Is there any way I can prove it?"

If you've already read the first 18 chapters of this book, you know that this caller has a lot to learn about herpes, starting with the fact that he probably can't be "sure" how he became infected at all. Partly for this reason, we prefer to focus on the medical and emotional implications of HSV. In fact, ASHA has found that lawsuits waged by one person against another over sexually transmitted infections often are pointless. Not only are they difficult to prove, such cases invade the privacy of both plaintiff and defendant, and can be a wrenching experience to the individuals involved. In addition, lawsuits tend to further stigmatize an infection that needs to be better understood and accepted by the general public.

Nonetheless, questions about herpes and the courts do come up from time to time, and ASHA has researched the issue with legal scholars so that we can provide factual answers on the subject.

COMMON LAW AND INFECTIOUS DISEASES

On the rise since the mid-1980s, lawsuits over sexually trans-mitted infections generally involve the principles of "common law" as opposed to "statutory law." Statutory law is usually the product of legislative bodies. Most of it is criminal law, includ-ing penalties such as jail sentences and fines, and the plaintiff in such cases is usually the federal, state, or local government. Since the HIV/AIDS epidemic began, for example, a number of states have passed laws that make it a crime to pass HIV to another person. In fact, the Ryan White Act of 1990, which provides emergency AIDS grants, requires states that receive these funds to make it a crime for HIV-infected people not to tell potential sex partners about their HIV status. Any violation of these laws would fall into the category of "statutory law."

"Common law," on the other hand, is generally not legislated but is based on a complex tradition of legal and moral principles as interpreted by the courts over time. And the plaintiff in such cases is usually an individual. Thus, if Jimmy wrongs Johnny, Johnny can sue, and it's up to the court to decide if Johnny is entitled to compensation. How do the courts make such deter-minations? They consider the arguments on both sides and refer to legal precedent within their state. As a result, the rules can vary quite a bit from one state to another.

People have long been held liable in common-law cases for exposing others to infectious diseases such as whooping cough and tuberculosis. In 1896, for example, the Wisconsin Supreme Court ruled that an employer should have told a servant that the employer's child was sick with typhoid fever before the servant cleaned the child's room. And in the 1920 case *Crowell* v. *Crowell*, the North Carolina Supreme Court held that a man was liable for fraudulently concealing from his bride that he had syphilis.

In the modern era, the same type of legal argument has been applied to infectious agents such as HIV, herpes simplex, and human papillomavirus. Because of its deadly consequences, lawsuits involving HIV infection have attracted greater publicity than other STD cases, but there have been some heavily hyped herpes cases as well.

Given the complex patchwork of local and state jurisdictions, no one knows how many STD cases are pending at any given time, but experts say that only a small percentage ever reach the courtroom.

THE LEGAL FRAMEWORK

If and when someone decides to launch a legal action, he or she generally pursues one of several common strategies. Some have sued on the grounds of "assault" or "infliction of emotional distress"; others on the basis of "fraud," "misrepresentation," or criminal "negligence."

Whatever the line of argument, however, these cases usually hinge on the issue of candor. Did the defendant know he or she had an STD? If not, did he or she take reasonable care to discover this condition? Did he or she withhold this information? And in doing so, did the defendant either accidentally or intentionally harm an innocent person?

While courts in various states might differ on the subtleties of interpretation in STD cases, a growing number of cases that have been settled so far is creating a legal consensus: A person has a right to know about the health of a sex partner. Thus, in the eyes of the law, individuals who have an STD have a duty to disclose this information to those with whom they're sexually intimate. If such a case goes to court, lying to conceal an STD is often considered a form of "intentional infliction" of harm. Simply failing to tell a partner about an STD, on the other hand, is more likely to be viewed as "negligence."

By the very nature of the supposed wrongdoing, these cases are difficult to prove. Things are said or not said—actions taken or not taken—in the heat of passion, and rarely are there witnesses.

In terms of physical evidence, the plaintiff often has a tough time establishing "causation"—proving that the defendant was the cause of the plaintiff's infection. With herpes, as we know, the infections may be acquired months or years before symptoms appear or are recognized. And more than half of all transmission occurs when a partner is asymptomatic or has symptoms but doesn't recognize them as herpes. If the plaintiff has had more than one partner, it may be impossible to prove that an infection came from a particular person. Pinpointing the source is—at the least—very difficult, and medical evidence must be supported by laboratory documentation of a first-episode HSV infection.

COMMON DEFENSES

Tracing the source of several other sexually transmitted infections can be equally challenging, so most defendants in STD cases avail themselves of expert opinion to challenge the proof of the claims made against them. As part of this process, the sexual past of the plaintiff often becomes an issue. Questions raised by the defense attorney will probably include the prior sexual history of the plaintiff and may well overstep our usual notions of privacy.

In addition, defense counsel in some of these cases have used strategies to question the very basis of the lawsuit. In some states, for example, it's a criminal offense ("fornication") for people to have sexual relations outside of marriage. In these states, the courts have sometimes ruled that a plaintiff cannot recover damages that occurred during an illegal act. Alternately, the defense will sometimes seek protection in laws that offer "spousal immunity," making claims between spouses a moot point.

While these continue to be used as defense strategies in some jurisdictions, the trend is to see them both as somewhat antiquated legal notions. In general, the courts have ruled that unmarried persons can sue their sexual partners, and California's *Kathleen K. v. Robert B.* set several precedents. The defendant argued that single people do not have a relationship of trust and confidence like married people, but the court ruled that intimate acts imply such a relationship. The defendant also argued that the plaintiff assumed the risk of getting an STD when she had intercourse. But the court said, essentially, that consent to intercourse is *not* consent to infection with an STD.

This last point is perhaps the most hotly contested in the legal arena. Some defense attorneys have been able to argue persuasively that anyone who has unprotected sexual intercourse in today's society, or who fails to ask about the sexual health of a partner, is equally responsible for infections that may be transmitted sexually, especially during a "one-night stand." In less casual relationships, however, the courts are more likely to see a lack of candor as a breach of trust.

Lawyers have found a great many subtleties in STD cases, and the legal landscape is still taking shape. There is, however, growing consensus about the importance of honest disclosure. If someone with an STD tells his or her partner in a meaningful way and gives the partner a choice about sexual involvement, grounds for legal action are vastly reduced. If, on the other hand, someone either conceals or lies about the infection, there is ample precedent to suggest he or she might be vulnerable in a legal action.

HERPES AND HEALTH INSURANCE

"When my wife recently decided to quit her job and start her own business, we had to abandon our old health insurance coverage," writes Steven. "But when we applied for family coverage from a new insurance carrier, they flagged my medical history because I'd had genital herpes. Can they legally deny us coverage?"

Slightly more common than questions about lawsuits are concerns about health insurance and the potential for discrimination. Overall, the news here is good. For nearly two-thirds of Americans covered under a group plan as part of their employee benefits, herpes generally is no issue at all. Millions of people with genital HSV routinely submit claims for office visits, prescription medication, and sometimes counseling. There may be limits placed on coverage under any particular policy, but herpes is seldom, if ever, regarded as different from other medical conditions.

Problems do sometimes emerge, however, for people who seek health insurance for themselves outside of large group plans. If you're applying for coverage as part of an individual or family plan, or as part of a small business plan with less than 25 participants, you probably will have to file a detailed application that may include questions about STDs. And for some insurers, a history of herpes or other sexually transmitted infections may prompt further questions.

As with large group policies, some small plans will regard herpes as a "pre-existing condition," just as they would in the case of many other illnesses. In this case, they would enroll you but would exclude herpes-related claims until some waiting period has passed. Others may accept you as a plan member but attach a "rider" to the policy that excludes coverage for herpes altogether.

There is also a small chance that your application to a small group may be rejected. In the late 1980s, for example, a few underwriters began to view any history of STDs as a "marker" for a much bigger risk—that of HIV infection.

While the "marker" theory is infuriatingly simplistic, people with herpes can take some comfort in the fact that this trend seems to be on the decline. Currently, most insurance companies examine individual or small group applications on a case-by-case basis and make decisions according to a variety of factors. Industry sources say that history of herpes alone would seldom be grounds for denying coverage. It's also important to remember that herpes claims have almost insignificant costs when compared with diabetes, heart disease, and many other ailments.

Anyone who has questions about health insurance or about discrimination in this area can take one of several steps:

- Work with an experienced, independent insurance
  agent who knows the insurance companies in your state

and can provide a list of companies that accept people with genital herpes.

• Consumers can contact the A.M. Best Company for annually updated ratings of life and health insurers. (Ratings reflect the financial stability of these companies.) A.M. Best can be reached at (908) 439-2200.

• Currently, some states have "open enrollment programs" in which applicants cannot be denied coverage for medical reasons. Your state department of insurance will have detailed information about these.

• Those who have problems getting coverage can appeal the company's decision in writing. We know of several cases in which the original decision was overturned solely on the basis of consumer protest. You also have the legal right of access to your Medical Information Bureau file, which insurers routinely review as part of their "credit check" on individual policies. This bureau, set up originally to root out fraudulent claims, keeps files on only a small percentage of insured individuals. The address: Medical Information Bureau, P.O. Box 105, Essex Station, Boston, MA 02112. Records will be sent to you or your physician for review.

RESOURCE LIST

ASHA SERVICES AND MATERIALS

The National Herpes Hotline (NHH) operates Monday through Friday, 9 AM to 7 PM Eastern Time. Information specialists are available to address questions related to diagnosis, transmission, prevention, and treatment of herpes simplex virus. The NHH also counsels individuals regarding emotional issues such as self-esteem and telling a partner, and provides referrals to local support groups and clinics. Call (919) 361-8488.

The ASHA Resource Center operates Monday through Friday, 9 AM to 6 PM Eastern Time. Callers can receive free brochures on herpes, and find out more about ASHA publications and services. Call (800) 230-6039.

To order or find out more about any of the following materials or services, please call the numbers listed above, visit ASHA's website at http://www.ashastd.org, or write:
ASHA/HRC
P.O. Box 13827
Research Triangle Park, NC 27709-3827

THE HELPER. Now in its 20th year, this quarterly journal covers herpes simplex virus (HSV) topics ranging from symptoms to psychosocial issues to treatment options. Each issue updates

INFORMATION ON MEDICATIONS

United States Food and Drug Administration (FDA) Office of Consumer Affairs: (301) 827-4420

Mailing address:
FDA HFE-88
5600 Fishers Lane
Rockville, MD 20857

As an alternative, the FDA Center for Drug Evaluation and Research handles inquiries from the public about approved medications: (301) 827-4573

Mailing address:
CDER, Executive Secretariat
HFD-8, FDA
5600 Fishers Lane
Rockville, MD 20857

Chiron Vaccines
Herpes Division
4560 Horton St.
Emeryville, CA 94608
Corporate Communications: (510) 923-2961

Glaxo Wellcome, Inc.
3030 Cornwallis Road
Research Triangle Park, NC 27709

Consumer Response Center: (800) 722-9292
8:00 AM - 5:30 PM, ET, M-F

Financial Assistance for Medications: (800) 722-9294
8:00 AM - 9:00 PM, ET, M-F

SmithKline Beecham
Pharmaceutical Division
One Franklin Plaza
P.O. Box 7929
Philadelphia, PA 19101
(800) 366-8900, Ext. 5231 or (215) 751-4000, Ext. 5231

OTHER RESOURCES

For support and counseling:
American Association of Marriage and Family Therapists
1100 17th St., NW , 10th Floor
Washington, DC 20036
(202) 452-0109, 9 AM - 5 PM, ET, M-F
The Association provides information through the mail about therapists in your area. Referrals are for solution-oriented therapy/counseling.

For nutrition information:
American Dietetic Association
(800) 366-1655, 10 AM - 5 PM, ET, M-F
Registered dieticians will answer questions about food and nutrients. Callers may also listen to recorded messages dealing with different topics, such as exercise and its effect on weight loss. These are varied monthly.

For reproductive health/family planning questions:
Local Chapters of the Planned Parenthood Federation of America
For referrals: (800) 829-7732
Local Planned Parenthood chapters may provide sex education over the phone and free pamphlets for men and women.

For information about insurance companies:
A.M. Best Co.
(908) 439-2200, Ext. 5742
Provides financial stability ratings of approximately 1,500 insurers.

For information about alternative treatments:
Office of Alternative Medicine Clearinghouse
National Institutes of Health
P. O. Box 8218
Silver Spring, MD 20907
(888) 644-6226

GLOSSARY

ACUTE OR EPISODIC THERAPY: Use of medication to relieve symptoms or hasten healing for an individual herpes outbreak.

ANTIBODIES: Elements of the body's immune response, these substances circulate in the blood and in other bodily fluids to fight disease-causing microbes.

ANTIGEN: Any foreign substance in the body, such as a fragment of a virus, that triggers the immune system to respond with antibodies or other defenses.

ASYMPTOMATIC REACTIVATION, ASYMPTOMATIC SHEDDING: An event in which latent herpes simplex virus reactivates at the nerve root and travels to a skin surface or mucous membrane, yet causes neither signs nor symptoms of infection that can be readily identified by the patient or a medical professional.

ASYMPTOMATIC TRANSMISSION: The spread of virus from one person to another during a period of asymptomatic shedding.

AUTOINOCULATION: The spread of HSV from one part of the body to another. This can result when a person with active herpes deposits a significant amount of virus onto some other vulnerable part of the body—most often a mucous membrane.

CELL CULTURE: A diagnostic test for many kinds of viruses. In a cell culture for HSV, a swab of the patient's herpes lesion is placed in a dish containing normal skin cells to see if HSV will grow.

CELLULAR IMMUNE RESPONSE: The portion of the body's immune response that involves T-lymphocytes or other cells designed to fight an "antigen" or invading microbe.

DISSEMINATED INFECTION: A herpes infection that spreads over a wider than usual area of the body, frequently afflicting internal organs.

FIRST EPISODE: The body's first encounter with a particular type of herpes simplex, an event that often produces marked symptoms. There are two types of "first episodes." A *primary first episode* describes the symptoms that appear in the person who has never been infected with either HSV-1 or HSV-2 before. It's sometimes called a "true primary."

A *nonprimary first episode* describes the symptoms that occur in the person who has been infected first with one type of HSV and then later infected with the second. For example, a person who is infected with HSV-1 and then years later infected with HSV-2 can be said to have a "first episode" of HSV-2 when he or she first has symptoms.

GANGLION: A knot-like grouping of the nerves that serve a particular part of the body.

GENITAL HERPES: While "genital herpes" can cause symptoms in a variety of sites below the waist, the term is used to denote all HSV infection that is latent in the sacral ganglion, at the base of the spine.

HSV: Abbreviation for herpes simplex virus. HSV-1 denotes herpes simplex type 1, the usual cause of herpes around the mouth or face ("cold sores," "fever blisters"); HSV-2 denotes herpes simplex type 2, the usual cause of recurrent genital herpes.

HERPES ENCEPHALITIS: A rare severe illness that occurs when the brain becomes infected with HSV.

HERPES GLADIATORUM: The presence of herpes lesions on the body caused by HSV infection that is transmitted usually through the abrasion of skin in a contact sport, such as wrestling.

HERPES WHITLOW: The presence of herpes lesions on the fingers or toes.

HERPESVIRUS: Any one of eight known members of the human herpesvirus family: herpes simplex type 1; herpes simplex type 2; varicella zoster virus; Epstein-Barr virus; cytomegalovirus; human herpes virus type 6; human herpes virus type 7; human herpes virus type 8.

LATENCY: The phenomenon by which HSV can hide away in the nerve roots in an inactive state, only to reactivate and cause viral shedding and lesions again.

LESION: A very general term denoting any abnormality on the surface of the body, whether on the skin or on a mucous membrane. Includes sores, pimples, tumors, and more.

MENINGITIS: An inflammation of the meninges, the protective covering around the brain, usually accompanied by stiff neck and extra sensitivity to light. *Septic meningitis*, caused by bacteria, can be a serious condition and must be treated immediately. *Aseptic meningitis*, associated with viral infections such as HSV and other causes, generally resolves by itself.

OCULAR HERPES: Symptoms caused by herpes infection in the eyes.

ORAL-FACIAL HERPES: The presence of latent herpes simplex infection in the trigeminal ganglion, at the top of the spine. When reactivated, oral-facial herpes can cause symptoms anywhere on mouth or face—typically cold sores. Recurrent oral-facial herpes is caused almost exclusively by HSV-1.

POSTHERPETIC NEURALGIA: Residual pain after a recurrence in the area involved. This does not represent viral shedding and is not contagious. Usually this problem diminishes with time.

PRODROME: An early warning symptom of illness, prodrome for a genital herpes outbreak often involves an aching, burning, itching, or tingling sensation in the genital area, buttocks, or legs.

PRODRUG: A medication that must undergo chemical conversion in the body in order to change to its active form.

RECURRENCE: The presence of lesions caused by reactivation of HSV ("outbreak").

STD: Sexually transmitted disease—any infection that is acquired through sexual contact in a substantial number of cases.

SACRAL GANGLION: The nerve root at the base of the spine that serves as the site of latency in genital herpes infections.

SEROLOGY: A test that identifies the antibodies in serum (a clear fluid that is a component of blood).

SEROSTATUS: A determination, based on serology, of whether a person has antibodies to any particular microbe—for example, HSV-1 or HSV-2.

STEROIDS: A group of drugs, including corticosteroids and anabolic steroids, that affect metabolism.

SUBCLINICAL REACTIVATION: When herpes reactivates without causing any visible symptoms.

SYMPTOMATIC REACTIVATION: The presence of lesions or any other symptoms caused by reactivation of HSV; a "recurrence."

SYSTEMIC SYMPTOMS: Fever, headache, fatigue, or other symptoms of illness affecting the whole body, as distinguished from the surface lesions seen in a herpes recurrence.

TRANSMISSION: The spread of herpes from one person to another.

TRIGGER (FACTOR): Any biologic or behavioral event that influences latent HSV to reactivate.

TRUE PRIMARY EPISODE: A person's first infection with either type of HSV: a *primary first episode.* See "first episode."

VIRAL REPLICATION: The process by which a virus makes more copies of itself.

FURTHER READING

❀

OVERVIEW OF GENITAL HERPES

Benedetti, J., Corey, L., Ashley, R. "Recurrence Rates in Genital Herpes after Symptomatic First-Episode Infections." *Annals of Internal Medicine* 1994; 12: 847-54.

Benedetti, J., Zeh, J., Selke, S., Corey, L. "Frequency and Reactivation of Nongenital Lesions among Patients with Genital Herpes Simplex Virus." *American Journal of Medicine* 1995; 98: 237.

Brock, V.B., Selke, S., Benedetti, J., Douglas, J., Corey, L. "Frequency of Asymptomatic Shedding of Herpes Simplex Virus in Women with Genital Herpes." *JAMA* 1990; 263: 418-20.

Centers for Disease Control and Prevention, Division of STD Prevention. "Sexually Transmitted Disease Surveillance 1995." Atlanta: U.S. Department of Health and Human Services, Public Health Service, Sept. 1996.

Corey, L. "The Current Trend in Genital Herpes: Progress in Prevention." *Sexually Transmitted Diseases* (Supplement 2) Mar/Apr 1994; 21: S38-S44.

Corey, L. "Genital Herpes." *Sexually Transmitted Diseases*. Second Edition. Ed. K. Holmes. New York: McGraw-Hill, 1990: 392-6.

Corey, L., Adams, H., Brown, Z., Holmes, K. "Genital Herpes Virus Simplex Infections: Clinical Manifestations, Course, and Complications." *Annals of*

Academy of Sciences 1992; 89: 10552.

Levy, J. "Three New Human Herpesviruses (HHV6, 7, and 8)." *Lancet* 1997; 349(9051): 558-63.

Roizman, B. "The Family Herpesviridae: A Brief Introduction." *The Human Herpesviruses.* Ed. B. Roizman, R. Whitley, and C. Lopez. New York: Raven Press, 1993.

Spear, P. "Biology of the Herpesviruses." *Sexually Transmitted Diseases.* Second Edition. Ed. K. Holmes. New York: McGraw-Hill, 1990: 379-80.

Weller, T. "Varicella and Herpes Zoster: Changing Concepts of the Natural History, Control, and Importance of a Not-So-Benign Virus." *New England Journal of Medicine* 1983; 309(22): 1362-8.

Wolk, S. "The Nature and Diagnosis of Clinically Important Viruses." *Physician Assistant* Jun 1993: 23-24.

TRANSMISSION AND PREVENTION

Abesfeld, D., Thomas, I. "Cutaneous Herpes Simplex Virus Infection." *American Family Practice* 1991; 43(5): 1655.

Bryson, Y., Dillon, M., Bernstein, D., Radolf, J., Zakowski, P., Garratty, E. "Risk of Acquisition of Genital Herpes Simplex Virus Type 2 in Sex Partners of Persons with Genital Herpes: A Prospective Couple Study." *Journal of Infectious Diseases* 1993; 167: 942-6.

Centers for Disease Control and Prevention. "Update: Barrier Protection Against HIV Infection and Other Sexually Transmitted Diseases." *MMWR* 1993; 42(30).

Douglas, J., Corey, L. "Fomites and Herpes Simplex Viruses: A Case for

Nonvenereal Transmission?" *JAMA* 1983; 250(22): 3093-4.

Judson, F., Ehret, J., Bodin, G., Levin, M., Reitmeijer, C. "In Vitro Evaluation of Condoms with and without Nonoxynol 9 as Physical and Chemical Barriers Against Chlamydia trachomatis, Herpes Simplex Virus Type 2, and Human Immunodeficiency Virus." *Sexually Transmitted Diseases* 1989; 16(2): 51-54.

Koutsky, L., Ashley, R., Holmes, K., Stevens, C., Critchlow, C., Kiviat, N., Lipinski, C., Wolner-Hanssen, P., Corey, L. "The Frequency of Unrecognized Type 2 Herpes Simplex Virus Infections among Women: Implications for Control of Genital Herpes." *Sexually Transmitted Diseases* Apr/Jun 1990; 17(2): 90-94.

Mertz, G., Benedetti, J., Ashley, R., Selke, S., Corey, L. "Risk Factors for the Sexual Transmission of Genital Herpes." *Annals of Internal Medicine* 1992; 116: 197-202.

Mertz, G., Coombs, R., Ashley, R., Jourden, J., Remington, M., Winter, C., Fahnlander, A., Guinan, M., Ducey, H., and Corey, L. "Transmission of Genital Herpes in Couples with One Symptomatic and One Asymptomatic Partner: A Prospective Study." *Journal of Infectious Diseases* 1988; 157(6): 1169-77.

Mertz, G., Schmidt, O., Jourden, J., Guinan, M., Remington, M., Fahnlander, A., Winter, C., Holmes, K., Corey, L. "Frequency of Acquisition of First-Episode Genital Infection with Herpes Simplex Virus from Symptomatic and Asymptomatic Source Contacts." *Sexually Transmitted Diseases* Jan/Mar 1985; 12(1): 33-39.

Rooney, J., Felser, J., Ostrove, J., Straus, S. "Acquisition of Genital Herpes from an Asymptomatic Sexual Partner." *New England Journal of Medicine* 1986; 314(24): 1563.

Infection. A Multicenter Double-Blind Trial." *JAMA* 1988; 260(2): 201-6.

Mertz, G., Loveless, M., Levin, M., Kraus, S., Fowler, S., Goade, D., Tyring, S. "Oral Famciclovir for Suppression of Recurrent Genital Herpes Simplex Virus Infection in Women." *Archives of Internal Medicine* 1997; 157: 343.

Mindel, A., Carney, O., Freris, M., Faherty, A., Patou, G., Williams, P. "Dosage and Safety of Long-Term Suppressive Acyclovir Therapy for Recurrent Genital Herpes." *Lancet* 1988; 1(8591): 926-8.

Nahata, M. "Clinical Use of Antiviral Drugs." *Drug Intelligence and Clinical Pharmacy* 1987; 21(5): 399-405.

Nilsen, A., Aasen, T., Halsos, A., Kinge, B., Tjotta, E., Wikstrom, K., Fiddian, A. "Efficacy of Oral Acyclovir in the Treatment of Initial and Recurrent Genital Herpes." *Lancet* 1982; 2: 571-3.

Patel, R., Bodsworth, N., Wooley, P., Peters, B., Vejlsgaard, G., Saari, S., Gibb, A., Robinson, J., and the International Valacyclovir HSV Study Group. "Valacyclovir for the Suppression of Recurrent HSV Infection: A Placebo-Controlled Study of Once Daily Therapy." *Genitourinary Medicine* 1997; 73: 105-9.

Reichman, R., Badger, G., Guinan, M., Nahmias, A., Keeney, R., Davis, L., Ashikaga, T., Dolin, R. "Topically Administered Acyclovir in the Treatment of Recurrent Herpes Simplex Genitalis: A Controlled Trial." *Journal of Infectious Diseases* 1983; 147(2): 336-40.

Reichman, R., Badger, G., Mertz, G., Corey, L., Richman, D., Connor, J., Redfield, D., Savoia, M., Oxman, M., Bryson, Y., Tyrrell, D., Portnoy, J., Creigh-Kirk, T., Keeney, R., Ashikaga, T., Dolin, R. "Treatment of Recurrent Genital Herpes Simplex Infections with Oral Acyclovir: In a Controlled Trial." *JAMA* 1984; 251: 2103-7.

Sacks, S., Aoki, F., Diaz-Mitoma, F., Sellors, J., Shafran, S. "Patient-Initiated, Twice-Daily Oral Famciclovir for Early Recurrent Genital Herpes: A Randomized, Double-Blind Multicenter Trial." *JAMA* 1996; 276(1): 44-49.

Safrin, S. "Treatment of Acyclovir Resistant Herpes Simplex Virus in Infections in Patients with AIDS." *Journal of AIDS* (Supplement 1); 1992: S29-32.

Safrin, S., Crumpacker, C., Chatis, P., Davis, R., Hafner, R., Rush, J., Kessler, H., Landry, B., Mills, J., and other members of the AIDS Clinical Trials Group. "A Controlled Trial Comparing Foscarnet with Vidarabine for Acyclovir-Resistant Mucocutaneous Herpes Simplex in the Acquired Immunodeficiency Syndrome." *New England Journal of Medicine* 1991; 325(8): 551-5.

Sollie, E. *Straight Talk With Your Gynecologist: How to Get Answers That Will Save Your Life*. Hillsboro, OR: Beyond Words, 1992.

Spruance, S., Tyring, S., DeGregorio, B., Miller, C., Beutner, K., and the Valaciclovir HSV Study Group. "A Large Scale Placebo-Controlled, Dose-Ranging Trial of Peroral Valaciclovir for Episodic Treatment of Recurrent Herpes Genitalis." *Archives of Internal Medicine* 1996; 156: 1729-35.

Straus, S., Mindell, S., Takiff, H., Rooney, J., Felser, J., Smith, H., Roane, P., Johnson, F., Hallahan, C., Ostrove, J., Nusinoff-Lehrman, S. "Effect of Oral Acyclovir on Symptomatic and Asymptomatic Virus Shedding in Recurrent Genital Herpes." *Sexually Transmitted Diseases* Apr/Jun 1989; 16(2): 107-13.

Wachsman, M. "Focus on Famciclovir: Review of Its Use in Genital Herpes Simplex Virus Therapy." *Formulary* 1995; 30: 587.

Wald, A., Zeh, J., Barnum, G., Davis, G. "Suppression of Subclinical Shedding of Herpes Simplex Virus Type 2 with Acyclovir." *Annals of Internal Medicine* 1996; 124: 8-15.

Whitley, R., Gnann, J. "Acyclovir: A Decade Later." *New England Journal of Medicine* 1992; 327: 782-9.

Whitley, R., Middlebrooks, M., Gnann, J. "Acyclovir: The Past Ten Years." *Advances in Experimental Medicine and Biology* 1990; 278: 243-53.

TAKING CONTROL—THE EMOTIONAL ISSUES

Aral, S., VanderPlate, C., Magder, L. "Recurrent Genital Herpes: What Helps Adjustment?" *Sexually Transmitted Diseases* 1988; 15(3): 164-6.

Catotti, D., Clarke, P., Catoe, K. "Herpes Revisited: Still a Cause of Concern." *Sexually Transmitted Diseases* 1993; 20(2): 77-80.

Greenwood, V., Bernstein, R. "Coping with Herpes: The Emotional Problems." Washington, D.C.: The Washington Center for Cognitive-Behavioral Therapy, 1982.

VanderPlate, C., Aral, S. "Psychosocial Aspects of Genital Herpes Virus Infection." *Health Psychology* 1987; 6(1): 52-72.

WELLNESS AND ALTERNATIVE THERAPIES

Eisenberg, D., Kessler, R., Foster, C., Norlock, F., Calkins, D., Delbanco, T. "Unconventional Medicine in the United States: Prevalence, Costs, and Patterns of Use." *New England Journal of Medicine* 1993; 328(4): 246.

Griffith, R. "Success of L-Lysine Therapy in Frequently Recurrent Herpes Simplex Infection." *Dermatological* 1987; 175: 183-90.

Longo, D. "Psychosocial Treatment for Recurrent Genital Herpes." *Journal of Consulting and Clinical Psychology* 1988; 56(1): 61-66.

Rooney, J., Bryson, Y., Mannix, M., Dillon, M., Wohlenberg, C., Banks, S., Wallington, C., Notkins, A., Straus, S. "Prevention of Ultraviolet-Light-Induced Herpes Labialis by Sunscreen." *Lancet* 1991; 338(8180): 1419-22.

HERPES AND PREGNANCY

Andrews, E., Yankaskas, B., Cordero, J., Schoeffler, K., Hampp, S., and the Acyclovir in Pregnancy Registry Advisory Committee. "Acyclovir in Pregnancy Registry: Six Years' Experience." *Obstetrics and Gynecology* 1992; 79(1): 8.

Arvin, A., Hensleigh, P., Prober, C., Au, D., Yasukawa, L., Wittek, A., Palumbo, P., Paryani, S., Yeager, S. "Failure of Antepartum Maternal Cultures to Predict the Infant's Risk of Exposure to Herpes Simplex Virus at Delivery." *New England Journal of Medicine* 1986; 315(13): 796-800.

Baker, D. "Herpes and Pregnancy: New Management." *Clinical Obstetrics and Gynecology* 1990; 33(2): 253-7.

Binkin, N., Koplan, J. "The High Cost and Low Efficacy of Weekly Viral Cultures for Pregnant Women with Recurrent Genital Herpes: A Reappraisal." *Medical Decision Making* 1989; 9(4): 226-30.

Brown, Z., Benedetti, J., Ashley, R., Burchett, S., Selke, S., Berry, S., Vontver, L., Corey, L. "Neonatal Herpes Simplex Virus Infection in Relation to Asymptomatic Maternal Infection at the Time of Labor." *New England Journal of Medicine* 1991; 324(18): 1249-50.

Brown, Z., Selke, M., Zeh, J., Kopelman, J., Maslow, A., Ashley, R., Watts, H., Berry, S., Herd, M., Corey, L. "The Acquisition of Herpes Simplex Virus during Pregnancy." *New England Journal of Medicine* 1997; 337(8): 509-15.

Brown, Z., Vontver, L., Benedetti, J., Critchlow, C., Hickok, D., Sells, C., Berry, S., Corey, L. "Recurrent Genital Herpes in Pregnancy: Variation of Recurrence Rates by Trimester and Risk Factors Associated with Asymptomatic Viral Shedding." *American Journal of Obstetrics and Gynecology* 1985; 153: 24-30.

Cone, R., Hobson, A., Brown, Z., Ashley, R., Berry, S., Winter, C., Corey, L. "Frequent Detection of Genital Herpes Simplex Virus DNA by Polymerase Chain Reaction among Pregnant Women." *JAMA* 1994; 272: 792-6.

Hardy, K., Arvin, A., Yasukawa, L., Bronzan, R., Lewinsohn, D., Hensleigh, P., Prober, C. "Use of Polymerase Chain Reaction for Successful Identification of Asymptomatic Genital Infection with Herpes Simplex Virus in Pregnant Women at Delivery." *Journal of Infectious Diseases* 1990; 162: 1031-5.

Harger, J., Amortegui, A., Meyer, M., Pazin, G. "Characteristics of Recurrent Genital Herpes Simplex Infections in Pregnant Women." *Obstetrics and Gynecology* 1989; 73(3): 367-72.

Kulhanjian, J., Soroush, V., Au, D., Bronzan, R., Yasukawa, L., Weylman, L., Arvin, A., Prober, C. "Identification of Women at Unsuspected Risk of Primary Infection with Herpes Simplex Virus Type 2 during Pregnancy." *New England Journal of Medicine* 1992; 326(14): 916-20.

Randolph, A., Washington, E., Prober, C. "Cesarean Delivery for Women Presenting with Genital Herpes Lesions: Efficacy, Risks, and Costs. *JAMA* 1993; 270(1): 77.

Scott, L., Sanchez, P., Jackson, G., Zeray, F., Wendel, G. "Acyclovir Suppression to Prevent Cesarean Delivery after First-Episode Genital Herpes." *Obstetrics and Gynecology* 1996; 87(1): 69-73.

Stone, K., Brooks, C., Guinan, M., Alexander, E. "National Surveillance for Neonatal Herpes Simplex Virus Infections." *Sexually Transmitted Diseases* 1989; 16(3): 152.

Suarez, M., Briones, H., Saaevdra, T. "Buttock Herpes: High Risk in Pregnancy." *Journal of Reproductive Medicine* 1991; 36(5): 367-8.

Whitley, R., Arvin, A., Prober, C., Corey, L., Burchett, S., Plotkin, S., Staff, S., Jacobs, R., Powell, D., Nahmias, A., Sumaya, C., Edwards, K., Alford, C., Caddell, G., Soong, S., and the National Institute of Allergy and Infectious Diseases Collaborative Antiviral Study Group. "Predictors of Morbidity and Mortality in Neonates with Herpes Simplex Virus Infections." *New England Journal of Medicine* 1991; 324(7): 450-4.

THE BROADER SPECTRUM OF HSV INFECTION

Arvin, A., Prober, C. "Herpes Simplex Virus Infections." *Pediatrics in Review* 1992; 13(3): 110-1.

Belongia, E., Goodman, J., Holland, E., Andres, C., Homann, S., Mahanti, R., Mizener, M., Erice, A., Osterhold, M. "An Outbreak of Herpes Gladiatorum at a High-School Wrestling Camp." *New England Journal of Medicine* 1991; 325(13): 906-10.

Bergstrom, T., Vahlne, A., Alestig, K., Jeansson, S., Forsgren, M., Lycke, E. "Primary and Recurrent Herpes Simplex Virus Type 2-Induced Meningitis." *Journal of Infectious Diseases* 1990; 162: 327.

Deschenes, J., Seamone, C., Baines, M. "The Ocular Manifestations of Sexually Transmitted Diseases." *Canadian Journal of Ophthalmology* 1990; 25(4): 179.

Gill, J., Arlette, J., Buchan, K. "Herpes Simplex Virus Infection of the Hand." *American Journal of Medicine* 1988; 84: 89-91.

Klotz, R. "Herpetic Whitlow: An Occupational Hazard." *Journal of the American Association of Nurse Anesthetists* 1990; 58(1): 8-13.

Shaw, G., Langston, A. "Herpes Simplex Virus Encephalitis: The Need for Early Diagnosis." *North Carolina Medical Journal* 1986; 47(1): 17-18.

Taylor, P., Nozik, R. "The Patient with Conjunctivitis." *Hospital Medicine* 1992; 28(8): 24-46.

Whitley, R. "Herpes Simplex Virus Infections of the Central Nervous System: Encephalitis and Neonatal Herpes." *Drugs* 1991; 42(3): 409.

Whitley, R. "Herpes Simplex Viruses." *Virology*. Second Edition. Ed. B. Fields, D. Knipe, et al. New York: Raven Press, 1990: 1867-86.

DIAGNOSIS

Ashley, R. "Laboratory Techniques in the Diagnosis of Herpes Simplex Infection." *Genitourinary Medicine* 1993; 69: 174-83

Ashley, R. "Inability of Enzyme Immunoassay to Discriminate between Infections with Herpes Simplex Virus Types 1 and 2." *Annals of Internal Medicine* 1991; 115: 520.

Koutsky, L., Stevens, C., Holmes, K., Ashley, R., Kiviat, N., Critchlow, C., Corey, L. "Underdiagnosis of Genital Herpes by Current Clinical and Viral-Isolation Procedures." *New England Journal of Medicine* 1992; 326(23): 1533-9.

Verano, L., Michalski, F. "Comparison of a Direct Antigen Enzyme Immunoassay, Herpchek, with Cell Culture for Detection of Herpes Simplex Virus from Clinical Specimens," *Journal of Clinical Microbiology* 1995; 33(5): 1378-9.

OTHER STDS

Centers for Disease Control and Prevention. "An Evaluation of Surveillance for Chlamydia trachomatis Infections in the United States, 1987-1991." *MMWR* 1993; 42(SS3): 21-27.

Donovan, P. "Testing Positive: Sexually Transmitted Disease and the Public Health Response." New York: Alan Guttmacher Institute, 1993.

Institute of Medicine, Division of Health Promotion and Disease Prevention. *The Hidden Epidemic: Confronting Sexual Transmitted Diseases.* Eds. T. Eng and W. Butler. Washington DC: National Academy Press, 1996.

INDEX

communication, 93-94, 97-108, 118-119

condom use in, 129-132

long-term, 92-93

sexuality in, 88, 109-111, 117-123

transmission between monogamous partners, 121-123

telling new partners, 102-108

Replens®. *See* lubricants

Replicate. *See* viral replication

Rhinovirus. *See* virus/viruses

Risk factors. *See* transmission

Sacral ganglion, 10-11, 26-27, 35, 205. *See also* ganglion

Safer sex, 111-123. *See also* condoms, transmission (prevention)

Secrecy. *See* emotional issues

Self-destructive feelings. *See* emotional issues

Self-esteem. *See* emotional issues

Self-image. *See* emotional issues

Self-treatment. *See* treatment

Septic meningitis, 159-160, 204. *See also* complications

Serology, 169-172, 205. *See also* diagnosis/diagnostic tests

Serostatus, 170, 205. *See also* diagnosis/diagnostic tests

Sex life/sexuality, 88, 109-111. *See also* condoms, emotional issues, relationships, safer sex, transmission

Sex toys, 116-117

Sexual partners. *See* condoms, emotional issues, relationships, transmission

Sexually transmitted diseases (STDs), 2, 205

attitudes about, 2, 118

chlamydia, 179

communication to partner, 102-108

definition, 205

ectopic pregnancy, 180

genital warts (HPV), 116, 181

gonorrhea, 2, 180

health insurance, 192-194

hepatitis B, 181-182

HIV/AIDS, 2, 115, 182

HSV as precursor to, 184-185

legal issues, 187-192

national HIV/AIDS hotline, 183, 197-198

national STD hotline, 183, 197-198

pelvic inflammatory disease (PID), 180

prevalence of, 2-3, 110, 179, 182

prevention of, 111-117, 127, 183-184

syphilis, 2, 181

trichomonas vaginalis, 182

Shame. *See* emotional issues

Shingles, 6, 8, 36. *See also* virus/viruses (varicella zoster)

Sites of preference. *See also* HSV-1, HSV-2, symptoms